Carry Me

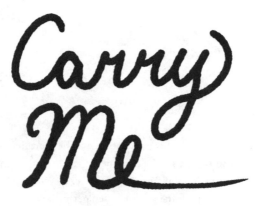

Carry Me

stories of pregnancy loss

Frieda Hoffman

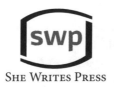

SHE WRITES PRESS

Published 2022
Printed in the United States of America
Print ISBN 978-1-64742-359-9
E-ISBN 978-1-64742-360-5
Library of Congress Control Number: 2021923634

For information, address:
She Writes Press
1569 Solano Ave #546
Berkeley, CA 94707

She Writes Press is a division of SparkPoint Studio, LLC.

All company and/or product names may be trade names, logos, trademarks, and/or registered trademarks and are the property of their respective owners.

Names and identifying characteristics have been changed to protect the privacy of certain individuals.

For anyone who's felt these pangs of grief

"Pain is important: how we evade it, how we succumb to it, how we deal with it, how we transcend it."

—Audre Lorde

"we all move forward when
we recognize how resilient
and striking the women
around us are"

—rupi kaur

CONTENTS

Introduction: Frieda

— *1* —

Chapter 1: Molly

"It's essential that we have other people."

— *15* —

Chapter 2: Desiree

"Feel what we feel and let it heal!"

— *24* —

Chapter 3: Ashley

"You don't have to be Wonder Woman."

— *32* —

Chapter 4: Suzy

"No baby, no client."

— *42* —

Chapter 5: Kari

"As a woman of color, I really expected more."

— *52* —

Chapter 6: Abby

"Nobody walks you through the finances of loss."

— *67* —

Chapter 7: Rae

"We remade our lives around this."

— 81 —

Chapter 8: Joanna

"I knew my babies were out there."

— 97 —

Chapter 9: Noreen

"You just end up quiet."

— 112 —

Chapter 10: Jackie

"I was entitled to feel a loss."

— 121 —

Chapter 11: Beth

"I needed to believe there was a greater purpose."

— 133 —

Chapter 12: Shirley

"Freeze your fucking eggs."

— 146 —

Chapter 13: Katie

"Life seems so much more fragile now."

— 158 —

Chapter 14: Miranda

"I can't believe it's still like this!"

— 172 —

Chapter 15: Deven
"We're transformers."
— 182 —

Chapter 16: Rose
"Bottom line is, we were killing him."
— 192 —

Chapter 17: Janice
"The assumption is pregnancy."
— 207 —

Chapter 18: KT
"The world needs our love!"
— 219 —

Chapter 19: Golda
"I love being a woman."
— 228 —

AUTHOR'S NOTE

I'D LIKE TO BE THE FIRST to acknowledge that my book is limited in scope with respect to exploring class, race, and ethnic disparities in pregnancy loss. There are only a few degrees of separation, at most, between me and the women I interviewed, a limiting factor that led to the majority of the voices in this work belonging to women like me: white, upper middle class, and cis-het. There is no doubt that the writing would be richer, more widely relatable, and of greater value to readers had I included more diverse voices. My ultimate failure to do so was not for want of trying.

As much as possible, I have tried to adopt the language of my interviewees and characters in these stories, particularly when it comes to capturing how they understand and discuss conception (baby vs. fetus, e.g.), whether they consider pregnancy to be singular or not ("I" vs. "we" got pregnant), etc., and their differing sociopolitical perspectives. I hope the inconsistencies aren't jarring.

Lastly, I have decided to change certain names to honor the requested anonymity of some protagonists or of their loved ones. Others were adamant about using their real names and boldly sharing their stories as part of their healing process. To each her own, with respect and gratitude.

INTRODUCTION

Frieda

THE INJECTIONS WEREN'T WORKING. My body wasn't working.

A week earlier, we had seen several follicles measuring in the *get-me-pregnant* zone on the ultrasound, which meant it was Go Time. Unfortunately, there seemed to be an inverse correlation between the dosing and my libido.

Lying on the exam table, a gel-capped wand gliding over my belly, I asked the nurse about side effects.

"Oh, honey," she said in between mumbled follicle measurements, "they're very common."

"I'm tired all the time. Constantly bloated. I have no sex drive whatsoever." As my eyes closed, I felt a cold tear slide down to my ear. "How are we supposed to have a baby like this? Is this normal?"

She smiled at me, then looked back at the screen. "The medication is making all these big, happy follicles—and lots of them, see?" She gestured with her head. "So your ovaries are blowing up like a balloon to make room for all those guys. That's the bloating."

"And what about the libido and exhaustion?"

1

"Well, isn't that just typical?" She turned to me with a raised eyebrow. "Can you imagine men doing any of this?"

No, I could not. I could scarcely imagine myself doing this much longer—cycling through hope and disappointment and adjusting meds, then hope and disappointment . . . I felt more like a petri dish than a fleshly woman with desires.

Joe and I were only four months into this fertility journey, and I was already starting to wonder whether it was time to pull the plug. The cumulative disappointment of not getting pregnant conspired with the mounting doubts I had about both my ability and my longing to conceive. I loved my freedom; I valued being able to pick up and go wherever, whenever. All those years of not wanting a child—then, BOOM, baby fever! Maybe it was as simple as hormones. What was I even doing here? The phrase that kept coming to mind was "square peg in a round hole."

My younger self could have seen this coming. As a vegetarian twentysomething, I vehemently opposed having kids because of the obvious threats of overpopulation. The youngest of three (four, really—I had a half-brother), I felt my parents had already done enough damage by out-spawning themselves. It didn't help that I had married a deeply cynical German who reveled in late-night discussions about Nietzsche and suicide, and had made it abundantly clear the summer we met that he never wished to be a father.

Things began to change shortly after the divorce. When those first hormonal tides washed their baby-craving waves over me I was in my early thirties, running a thriving cafe business, and dating someone who just might be marriage material.

My brother and his wife had just had their first baby, and I relished watching Frances. I'd strap on the Baby Björn sling and walk through their leafy Oakland neighborhood, cooing in her ear, playing with her tiny doll fingers, kissing her impossibly soft head. Mm . . . that intoxicating scent of baby!

Changing her diapers wasn't a chore, it was a love act. When she kicked and screamed, shaking her little fists in the air, I would wiggle my features into a silly face and sing her to a state of quiet calm. These mundane efforts felt like my womanly calling, my life's ultimate purpose. To be recognized by this perfect little peanut and see her angelic face light up for me, to make her laugh—was there anything more precious?

The baby fever extended to complete strangers. One day I watched a mother in a coffee shop, dressed like me and probably drinking the same hipster pour-over, as she danced with her baby daughter, who flopped about on a bistro table like a marionette, giggling and drooling with delight. This reverie was interrupted when I heard my own tears hit the pages of the journal I'd been writing in.

I was fevering so badly I fantasized about my older gay cousin and his partner as my baby-daddies. They were trying to figure out having a child of their own and had proposed helping me father mine.

I mulled over their offer. Did I want to be a single mother, albeit coparenting with my dear cousins? No. An emphatic *no*. I wanted romance. I wanted the magic of combining my DNA with that of the love of my life. I wanted my partner to worship my pregnant body and help deliver the baby. I wanted to peek through the bedroom door and see that baby's father snuggling with our child as he read him or her bedtime stories. I wanted us all to go camping, make s'mores, and stargaze from our shared tent. I craved that partner.

And now here I was with that partner, my fiancé, walking out of the fertility clinic and questioning our path forward.

We could continue with the injections for another few months or look into other options like intrauterine insemination (IUI) or *in vitro* fertilization (IVF), neither of which appealed to me. It became clear that I needed to stop or, at the very least, press pause. Give myself a break and an opportunity to process.

I made an appointment to see an old astro-therapist friend, who took one look at my horoscope and said, "Frieda, some women aren't meant to be mothers." Her comment would have crushed me weeks earlier, but now I took it as validation of the ambiguity and anguish I felt.

After discussing the change of heart with Joe, ever the quiet cheer-leader and supportive partner, I sank into possibility space—and my entire being relaxed. I would get my body back. And with my ovaries no longer in charge of scheduling, I would get my life back, too. Sex could be fun again. I wouldn't have to wonder if I would be a good mother or what I'd have to sacrifice to have a family. Joe and I would remain strong; we agreed we didn't need a child to chart a meaning-ful life together. I was more than ready to embrace this next chapter of "Not Trying" (subtitle: "Moving On").

Joe and I got married and bought a house, and I started a new real-estate venture. But the greatest achievement of 2016 may have been (drum roll, please) that I got my first natural period in fourteen years. The previous five years had been a series of failed attempts of reactivating my menstrual cycle after a decade of being on the pill and running a stressful business.

Joe and I joked about the expensive non-baby we had made with our fertility experiment, but maybe it was worth it to have finally woken up those ovaries that had pulled a Rip Van Winkle on me. At last, I felt like a woman again.

Not two years later, in April 2018, I had The Period From Hell. After a solid week of intense bleeding and clotting, I began to wonder if The Period might actually be something else. But if I was miscarrying, then I must have been pregnant. Was that even possi-ble? Despite the obvious evidence of increasingly regular menstrual cycles, I was still dubious about my ability to conceive, and that doubt stubbornly fed back into the possibility of miscarriage. Yet I wasn't entirely blind.

I went to see my friend Reba that afternoon. She was her usual mix of cheery and crazed. After dancing about and clearing clutter from her office table, she sat down across from me.

"Whew, that was a day!" she exclaimed, bursting into that infectious Reba grin. "Sooo . . ." She leaned toward me, letting out a long sigh. "How have you been?"

I choked up. Words weren't forming.

"Oh, dear. You've had a day too." She handed me a tissue.

Right on cue, I began sobbing.

I had no idea I was holding so much tension and emotion around the pregnancy and what I was only now starting to grasp as my loss. There was no denying it anymore. How clichéd it felt to finally get pregnant once the urgency to make a baby had fizzled out. I'd rolled my eyes at so many friends and relatives who'd told me it would happen that way. "Just relax with all this fertility stuff. Go on a vacation, forget about it, and next thing you know . . ." I didn't believe it then, and I don't imagine it magically happens like that now. Still, I felt duped by some perverse higher power.

All the dust that had settled was kicked back up now. Did this mean we should be trying again? We had just started high-fiving each other over our DINKs (Double Income No Kids) status. We were enjoying our life—taking risks, starting new ventures, traveling. Now that we knew it was possible, should we reconsider?

Ultimately, we chose to stay on our path and enjoy the childfree life we were building for ourselves. We still weren't using protection. I figured if I had miscarried without knowing I was pregnant, it was unlikely my body would carry another pregnancy.

Joe and I went through a rocky phase around our two-year anniversary and started seeing a couples therapist. Despite our moments of celebrating life without kids, a part of me felt estranged in the relationship without the shared goal of parenthood.

Around this time, I began to notice subtle changes in my body. I was tender, more sensitive to smell, and especially prone to crying.

My hips swelled. My breasts suddenly burst out of my bra. I went into a CVS and almost bought a pregnancy test but ended up with a bag of makeup I still haven't worn. I told myself it was just the relationship stress. I was probably overeating and not getting enough exercise.

The next day, I bought a test and a bar of chocolate. I peed on the stick, and immediately both lines appeared bright blue.

I had to double-check the instructions to make sure I was reading it right. My heart pounded. I took a few deep breaths and went out to share the news.

When I presented the stick to Joe, he broke into a smile and pulled me close. "Babe! Congratulations?" he asked.

"It's so crazy," I said, my fingernails clawing at my pants leg. "Can you believe it?"

"I know!" he said, his green eyes welling up. "But I knew something was up. Your tits, geez!"

We laughed, wiping away tears.

My phone buzzed in my pocket. It was my bestie calling from abroad. She shrieked her congratulations through WhatsApp's compressed line before admonishing me to get back to talking with my husband. Before we hung up, I confessed, "I'm so confused . . . but it's like I finally have this affirmation of my womanhood."

She immediately rebuked me. "Frie, you were just as much of a woman before, whether or not you could have a baby. Don't make it about gender." I realized I had been conflating these things all along, and I hated myself for it.

I became stuck in an ambiguous space. The timing was awful. Could our relationship survive having kids? Would a baby bring us closer together? What ever happened to rejoicing in our DINKsdom?

The next morning, I ran into an old friend on my way to work. I immediately shared the news, along with my doubts about mothering and the viability of the pregnancy. I didn't mention that Joe and I weren't in a great place.

"Aw, man," he gushed, shaking his head. "I just can't wait to see your belly get all big!"

Hugging him good-bye, I felt a pang in my heart. *Right. If it ever gets big.* I walked on, dabbing away tears of joy and anxiety, and decided to stop telling people I was pregnant.

My ambivalence gave way to problem-solving, leaving no positive or certain prognosis, which led me back to ambivalence. I couldn't have been more than five or six weeks pregnant, but I knew I was farther along than I'd made it with the last pregnancy. At thirty-eight, with a history of fertility issues, my chance of miscarrying was not only high but also indifferent to whether we wanted the baby or not. If we decided we weren't ready to have a child, and acknowledged we might never be, we would have to choose to change course—an impossible decision. Round and round I went, deliberating.

Joe experienced his own mix of emotions. At one point, he admitted he was unsure he could commit to the task of fatherhood. I felt an overwhelming fear of being left alone to care for our child and worried that my resentment, if not the imbalance alone, would ruin our relationship.

Moments later, we gazed into each other's eyes and imagined cuddling and dancing with our little munchkin. What if this was our only chance?

Only four days in and acknowledging the impossibility of the situation, we decided to wait another week and see how we felt.

Getting ready for bed that night, I noticed some pains. Soon they became unbearable and entirely unfamiliar: deep, shooting pangs in my lower left abdomen; what felt like a pole being jabbed into my anus and rear vaginal walls; cramping throughout my pelvis. I barely slept.

The next day, the doctor didn't see anything on the ultrasound and was concerned the pregnancy could be ectopic, with the fetus stuck in a fallopian tube or elsewhere outside the uterus, so she sent me to radiology for a more thorough exam. From there, I was transferred to the emergency room.

A nurse invited me to lay down before shuffling off. Exhaustion and confusion sank in as I sat on the edge of the gurney. My body seemed impossibly heavy for how hollow I felt. Joe held up the sheets for me while I climbed in, slow and shivering.

"We just need to run a few more tests to know what's going on here," said a friendly voice. A doctor poked his head into the room. "Can I get you some more blankets?"

"Thanks," I said, nodding.

Joe caressed my hand while I held my belly and cried quiet tears. A nurse came in and hooked me up to an IV. After a grueling series of attempts to find an adequate vein, she drew blood from my other arm and brought me heating pads for the cramping.

An hour later, a new doctor—bearing a speculum—introduced herself. Oh god.

"Is this a desired pregnancy?" she asked. Yet another doctor appeared.

"Um. No?" I offered. "I mean, it wasn't planned but . . ."

"We just have to ask." As she examined me, she gently explained their concerns. "We've gotten most of your labs back and there's no conclusive evidence that this is ectopic, but the lateralized pain suggests it may be. You're most likely miscarrying."

I nodded as the speculum slid out and my body relaxed.

Their main concern, echoed by the radiology doctor, was internal bleeding from a ruptured fallopian tube. Another possibility was that I wouldn't pass the fetal tissue on my own, in which case they'd have to induce an abortion with the aggressive chemotherapy drug methotrexate and do a dilation and curettage (D&C) to scrape the womb clean.

Cramping throughout the discussion of these less-than-savory options, I desperately hoped my body would rally and let go of the pregnancy naturally. I lamented the prospect of having to take cancer meds to abort a fetus we had longed for two years ago but was now stuck in the wrong place at the wrong time. All the while, I felt the sting of losing the opportunity to have a baby—our baby.

When we left the hospital that night, it was clear that something much graver was happening outside of our little orbit. The air was thick with smoke, our eyes burning as we walked back to the car. In the ER, we'd heard chatter amongst the nurses about a fire northeast of the Bay Area. We didn't know then how tragic the news was or how extensive the effects for the surrounding areas would be.

Over those next few days, ash from the deadly Camp Fire began to blow over from Butte County and settle over the Bay. The cramping continued and the bleeding intensified.

Joe drove me to the beach, and though it was cold and smoky, I ambled slowly up the coastline. Walking back to the dunes, a pack of elephant seals swam alongside me, throwing their slick, dark bodies in the air. Uncertainty prevailed, but those playful creatures offered some reassurance that things would be okay. I would have to be calm and let the waves of life wash over me.

I hadn't told anyone yet, not even my mom. I knew I should reach out, but I felt too dark. I didn't want anyone to have to bear my burden. I looked online for support around the ever-changing physical symptoms and was shocked at how little was out there. I didn't want WebMD or some random lady's frenzied blog post. I had no stomach for reading about God's will or how my child would be waiting for me up in Heaven. Where were regular women with real experiences and wisdom?

I canceled plans, making up excuses each time, and felt irresponsible for doing so, like I was somehow a slacker for having a miscarriage.

Five days into the cramping and bleeding, my pregnancy hormone (HCG) levels were falling but still deemed problematic, given the likely ectopic nature of the pregnancy. Even so, I felt certain the worst of it was over. Plus, as weak as I was physically, I still had my emotional restlessness to contend with, so I did what I usually do when I'm anxious: I went for a walk.

It was a mild fall day, but I bundled up in my winter jacket. Setting out, I had to remind myself to slow down. Would I hurt myself from overexertion? It was Sunday, not the time to call my Ob/Gyn. I opted for a pep talk instead.

Breathe deeply into your diaphragm—I inhaled—*and out through your mouth.* I exhaled. *Allow yourself to relax completely.*

I felt a dark hollowness at my core; my cheeks were wet and warm. I'd never felt so sad or so alone in my sadness.

You were a woman before, without a period, and you're a woman now, without a baby. I repeated this a few times, willing it to burn itself into my brain. *You may not be as physically or emotionally strong as you would like, but you will get stronger. You'll take care of yourself*—breathing into my diaphragm—*and love yourself*—exhaling audibly. *You will share the wisdom that comes from this incredibly painful experience.*

Our home in Berkeley looked more apocalyptic by the day with the fires still raging: ash-dusted cars and trees, people in respirators and makeshift masks, schools closed, no kids in sight. The Air Quality Index (AQI) had reached over 300 in some parts of the Bay. I was exhausted from the miscarriage and increasingly worse conditions at home, catastrophic events unfolding both within and around me.

The trip up the coast we'd booked months earlier promised cleaner air, rest, and recovery. The AQI wasn't much lower in Bodega Bay, however, so we largely stayed indoors. I continued to bleed and cramp, but the physical symptoms were subsiding. Since the air hadn't improved back home and my doctors were satisfied enough with my progress report to skip the blood work, we continued north for another few days.

In a rented room at a stranger's place on the Sonoma Coast, eleven days after leaving the hospital, the cramping suddenly returned. It was nearly midnight.

I wailed in agony as Joe asked me where the pain was on a scale from one to ten, a whiff of irritation in his voice.

It was an eight. No amount of ibuprofen, CBD oil, or deep breathing could quell the pain.

Joe massaged my back for a while, then fell asleep. I knew he was reaching his limit, and I felt guilty for adding onto his stress.

I woke the next morning to find my pajama bottoms damp and red. I sighed and tossed my underwear in the trash bin. At least the cramping had stopped.

Days later, the gushing became a trickle and my HCG levels finally bottomed out. After another few weeks, I was able to sleep on my left side again.

Then came the hospital bill—over $3,000, despite having health insurance—and the slow crawl out of isolation into healing.

Even with my background in social work and psychology, I struggled to reach out to close friends and relatives. I sat on the couch and listened to moody women croon through the stereo speakers, an endless pot of steeping herbs and a stack of magazines beside me. I took countless meditative walks in the leafy hills and at the dog park by the shore. I found myself pacing our small backyard and pulling young weeds after the rain, my core still sore and tender from the cramping.

Finally, I began opening up to friends and family—including my mother, who suddenly remembered that she, too, had suffered a miscarriage before my oldest brother was born. The more I shared, the more I understood that I was not alone. The empathy from others came flooding in, along with a resounding chorus of "Me too" and "I'm here if you want to talk."

But why weren't we talking about it in the first place? Why wasn't there a conversation or support group I could easily jump into and share my experience? Why did I and so many others know so little about pregnancy loss? The emotions whirred around for another few months before culminating in the birth of this project—a release valve that had a greater purpose than self-soothing or catharsis.

I set out to write a book to create the resource I wished I'd had around the time of my loss. Only after sharing my story with others did I realize that I wasn't alone, either in my experience or in my desire for such a resource.

Why had I felt so alone? It seemed so many people were coming forward with their own stories of loss. All I'd needed to do was say something; with that, others suddenly had the permission they'd apparently needed in order to share with me. As I heard their stories, I learned just how many women believe they are alone and indeed suffer alone—paradoxically, given how widely shared the experience of pregnancy loss is.

Carry Me brings everyday women's experiences of pregnancy loss to light so we can feel more connected to one another, deepen our understanding, and better care for ourselves and others. Through my own journey and those of the courageous women who've shared their stories in these pages, I've set out to discover what we can learn and how we might apply those lessons to improve the experiences of those suffering the fallout of pregnancy loss.

The title is inspired by a sisterhood of support and bearing witness that became evident in my interviews. The message I took from each of these conversations was: *Carry me, and I will carry you.* These stories share a sense of strength and resilience intrinsic to the many challenges and transformations of being a woman, including pregnancy loss. Together, through the sharing of resources, wisdom, and stories, our strength is magnified.

As I began to write, I became more aware of my heightened vulnerability. There was still so much to know and process. Would I be childless forever? Could my life be as fulfilling and meaningful without biological children? Would I ever be truly at peace with a childfree life? Could my marriage survive it, or even be stronger for it?

Most people want to move past their loss and go back to their regular lives—try again, focus on the family they have, find their new normal. I, however, have decided to stay in this slurry of loss and love. I've learned that my vulnerability in sharing and asking the tough questions is essential—not only for my own processing and healing but for others' as well.

Carry Me illustrates that women's experiences of pregnancy loss are fundamentally human. Miscarriage and stillbirth encompass far more than the relegation "women's issue" allows us to appreciate. They touch on trauma, grieving, and the politics of women's bodies. And while pregnancy loss is very much in the domain of women's health, it's also a public-health issue of awareness and education.

The statistic most often cited regarding miscarriage is one in four[1]. But according to some estimates, when the losses that go unreported or remain unknown to women because of early termination are accounted for, that number increases to up to one in three[2]. That's over three million pregnancy losses per year in the US alone—losses that affect not just the mothers but also their partners and support networks. Nearly everyone knows somebody affected by pregnancy loss, yet we're not comfortable—as a society, or even in the relative safety of the company of friends and sisters—discussing this serious and prevalent health issue.

It's time to break the silence.

I wrote this book to serve as a resource for the women and partners experiencing pregnancy loss, the public health experts and care providers who hope to better understand and support them, and the larger readership interested in how such adversity and loss can strengthen and transform us.

I've chosen to focus on the unique stories and people rather than statistics, though I have woven in some figures in order to provide contextual understanding. I've drawn on real women's accounts to highlight strikingly different experiences of miscarriage and still-birth, as well as the related challenges of infertility, finances, relationship dynamics, healthcare and recovery, grieving, and resilience.

In sharing these stories, I hope to create meaning and solace for readers, and help normalize the dialogue around pregnancy loss and grief so that others don't have to suffer alone.

We are not alone.

CHAPTER 1

Molly

"It's essential that we have other people."

MOLLY WAS KNEE-DEEP IN TOMATOES, her fingertips covered in a sticky tar of vines and dirt. The rich soil of a lush Kansas summer, crashing thunderstorms, and endless sunshine had summoned a garden that was nearly redder than it was green.

She moved slowly, methodically, harvesting dozens of pounds of ripe fruit to dry. The kitchen counter was a mess of seed, skin, and juice. As she wiped the pulp-stained seeds from her elbows, Molly thought about fertility and the cycle of life. Her own fertility and spring's fallow fate.

Her body froze with the memory.

Angered mourning dissolved into hushed wonder as she delivered the tiny pouch in the toilet with an unceremonious plop. Earlier she'd been all fiery fury. "You just get to ejaculate, but I have to go through all of this shit!" she'd barked at Peter. Now she embraced her inner scientist: She pulled the little peach of a sac from the enamel bowl and gently rotated it in her hand. Then she opened it carefully with her thumb and, as amniotic fluid pulsed outward, observed the rice-size grain that would have been her baby.

"I was so blown away by the beauty," Molly told me, walking in her white bobble hat and mittens on a brisk winter morning. "This moment where it had paused and lived in my body. And then it was in my hand."

Molly carried the fetus outside and pointed to a tree in a grove of great pines on Peter's sprawling property. He dug a hole in the dirt, and they offered their thanks as Molly returned the breathtaking form to the earth.

"I hadn't thought any of it out, I was kind of on autopilot mode," she said. "But it was amazing."

By then, Molly had been on autopilot for a while.

Peter wasn't the man she'd fallen in love with just two years before. That was Tyler, the free-spirited twenty-four-year-old she'd met wrapping up her doctoral studies in psychology. She was thirty-three at the time, and though they'd hit it off spectacularly, he wasn't making any moves in her direction; he seemed to be on his own, much younger path.

Reluctantly, Molly decided to move on.

She went back to Kansas, where she did her clinical internship and met Peter, a massage therapist for athletes at Kansas State. He was kind-hearted and giving. They trusted one another. But there was no equilibrium: Peter was smitten with her, while she was only lukewarm about him. But her hormones were acting up, and she was starting to fixate on having a baby.

Their relationship was on and off due to differences they could never reconcile. Molly came from a highly educated, upper-middle-class family; Peter had working-class roots. She wanted to explore and live large, while he was content to stay in the Midwest and make himself smaller.

Molly leveled with herself. She'd already had several serious relationships, and nobody had measured up to her standards. Perhaps they were unreasonable; maybe her expectations were too high. Meanwhile, life was getting on. Plus, she couldn't ignore the rising baby fever within her.

"We had a three-day window around my ovulation, so we figured let's have sex. Not trying, per se," she explained, "but I said the words, and he was all about it."

She was on a solo work trip in Chicago when she missed her period. The Windy City had always been a bad omen for Molly, a place of uncanny doom and disaster. She was staying at someone's flat who wasn't even her friend, and was teary and anxious with the news of her pregnancy. She could barely sleep.

"I was hit with this terror," Molly recalled. "The fact that I was in Chicago—this thunderous darkness came over me. I thought, 'My god, if I am pregnant, I'm getting an abortion.' I just didn't want to be with this person."

Knowing in her bones and in her womb the loneliness she would feel if she remained in the relationship, Molly felt profoundly alone. Yet she longed to be a mother.

Once she got back to Kansas and felt Peter's warmth and serenity, she was able to calm her nerves. It would all work out, she told herself.

Soon she was swept up in the vision of a home birth and an enchanted life on all that beautiful, meditative land. They chose a midwife, and Molly shared the news with a coworker and her little sister Ann, both pregnant at the time.

Molly embraced the good fortune of her pregnancy. She'd always had an obsession with birth. She'd seen several friends through their deliveries as a doula. Now she could barely contain the excitement of her own swelling belly and journey into motherhood.

It was a Saturday, just shy of eleven weeks, when Molly felt an ominous vise grip at her uterus. Her hips and thighs swelled and she had some spotting but, it being the weekend, she couldn't get in touch with her doctor to gauge how concerned she ought to be. It was a long drive to the nearest hospital. Her midwife, when she finally reached her, was dismissive; it was still too early in the pregnancy to say one way or the other, she said. But she advised Molly to get an ultrasound anyway.

Molly's mother drove her to a 4D ultrasound booth in a strip mall outside of town. The technician moved the wand over her belly, but there was no heartbeat. Nothing. Just a ghost of her dreams.

For days after the burial, Molly bled heavily. The thick, crimson clumps reminded her of raw cutlets of beef. She was shocked by how much of her own body she had passed.

"For a long time, I didn't talk to anybody," Molly said. "Never had anything measured or checked out. I spoke with the midwife once." She wiped her red nose with the back of a mitten. "I was just so on my own."

Molly hadn't been in touch with her doctor since her first well visit, and nobody bothered to follow up after she miscarried.

Her neighbor, a family doctor, came by the house about a week later. He'd been hunting on the land and popped in to ask how Molly was doing with the pregnancy. She told him about her loss, that she'd been home all day grieving. With his little daughter on his shoulders, her pink cowboy boots resting on his chest, he told Molly that only one in 300 fertilized eggs ever makes it to a baby.

"It's actually quite hard to have a healthy baby," he said. "People just don't know the odds."

Molly felt comforted by his presence and his words. The tangible science, along with the inexplicable miracle of life and death, stirred inside her.

She shared with me that her cousin had recently had a baby at forty-five after trying IVF unsuccessfully three years earlier. "Out of nowhere, got pregnant and had a healthy baby. Just like that!" She smiled at me with damp blue eyes. "We have to surrender to the mystery. That's one thing I am entirely sure of."

Besides her neighbor's brief visit, Molly self-isolated. She felt closed off from her sister Ann and her mother, for both of whom the weight of Molly's miscarriage was too great to bear. She didn't feel she could lean on Ann, who was still joyfully expecting.

This unwanted yet common side effect of loss presents a difficult reality for women struggling to cope: their pain makes pregnant women and new moms feel like they can't enjoy their successful pregnancies. The effect, Molly told me, is that women who've lost their pregnancies feel even more awful and alone.

Molly was in her early teens when her mother got together with her stepdad. They wanted to have a baby of their own, but her mother was already in her early forties. Over the course of two years, she had five miscarriages. Decades later, Molly felt her mother was still emotionally unresolved about her losses. Although she craved compassion and support, she felt she had to protect her mother from the sadness and emotions triggered by her own miscarriage.

Molly realized that the only solace she would find was from other women who'd lost a pregnancy. Others' support felt empty.

"For a couple of months, I craved being around women who'd had miscarriages," she said, shaking her head. "I wanted nothing to do with anyone else. Literally no one else. Like, 'Fuck off, you don't understand, go away.'"

Molly's grief had moved from initial shock and denial into anger. She was desperate to connect with other women to help process her loss, to commiserate, but also to reach some kind of acceptance.

As a psychologist and someone who's dealt with loss firsthand, Molly feels our society is ill-equipped to deal with grief. Our modern culture undervalues intentional space and ritual ceremony for processing grief and its attendant feelings.

"We need to have a space to talk about it—space to celebrate but also respect perspectives, respect this as a thing that can happen in women's lives," Molly stressed. "Normally, it's just brushed under the rug."

Bearing witness to grief and trauma is the key, she said, to unlocking ourselves to the healing process. The act of witnessing the powerful emotions that move through us as we grieve can bring people together and help us grow and heal faster.

A few weeks before I met Molly, she'd attended a grief ceremony based on the spiritual teachings of Sobonfu Somé, who passed away in 2017. She was of the Dagara people of Burkina Faso, whose grief rituals play an integral role in community connection and healing. Somé and her husband had a vision that Westerners needed to learn these rituals, because they were out of touch with their grief and it was causing them to destroy the world.

In her own clinical work, Molly saw that repressed feelings often festered and became bigger problems like depression, shame, guilt, anger, and disconnection.

"It's essential that we have other people," Molly said. "Because you can cry, and I can cry about my miscarriage, cry about feeling like a failed woman. But something doesn't happen if nobody loves me through it in that moment." She stopped walking and turned to me. "We need to be seen, and then we can turn around and do it for someone else."

Molly was touching on the symbiosis of being seen and bearing witness. Once we have opened ourselves up and shared our losses and our traumas, we can then hold space for others who are grieving and carry them through it.

According to researchers at Columbia University and the Dulwich Centre, the most difficult stories we so often keep to ourselves lead to significantly faster healing and greater overall well-being when we relay them to others. In fact, simply hearing someone else's story conveys similarly strong psychological and physiological benefits[3].

"Grief comes in waves," Molly explained. "It comes and then it's gone. And we're there on the shore. We don't know how we got here, but the wave got us here, and so now I can hold space for you."

Molly's own experience of grief revealed another facet of pregnancy loss: silence begets silence. Molly felt the internalized shame of having a miscarriage turn into silence that then communicated unconsciously to other woman that they too should be silent. In her eyes, women do a great disservice to other women—and partners, families, et al—by not breaking the silence to speak their messy truths and sorrows.

"It's terrible," she groaned. "Like, I'm going to crawl into a hole and suffer by myself, and that's what you should do if it happens to you. That's the message, whether we intend it or not."

I was curious what else had helped Molly out of her grief and isolation.

"Time," she answered, gazing off toward the San Francisco Bay. "And my sister."

Molly was out hiking with her sister when Ann suddenly grabbed her arm and turned to her.

"Look me in the eyes," she pleaded. "Don't marry him, you're not happy. He's not your person."

It was a bold thing for anyone to say, but especially for her little sister. And Molly knew she was right. She'd sensed it in Chicago when she learned she was pregnant.

"I had such an intense rippling and ricocheting through my body in that moment," she said. "I feel like that actually caused the miscarriage."

There was something strangely empowering for Molly about realizing that some part of her had heard the call to have a baby, but another part had known it was neither the right time nor the right person. Her body's intuition gave her a renewed sense of awe for life.

When Molly first met Tyler, who she couldn't feel more 'Yes!' about, she instinctively knew he was her match. Years later, after leaving Peter and her life in Kansas, Molly still felt magnetically drawn to Tyler. She was thirty-seven.

Tyler, twenty-eight, told her he might have to go to the Himalayas to sit in a cave for a couple of years because he was still exploring life. Molly chuckled at the memory, but she understood. They both wanted to live expansively and mutually support one another in this aim. He could go to the mountains, she could plant heirloom tomatoes. They could each explore the world in their own right— she trusted that they could have it all. She certainly hoped that this would include motherhood.

"Once we got together, I was really ready to have a baby," she said, laughing.

When she found out she was pregnant with Tyler's child, a radiant calm washed over her. Molly was sure, with a quiet kind of knowing, that it would be a boy. They decided to marry just before their son, Theo, now three and a half, was born.

With Tyler, Molly never doubted the health or viability of her pregnancy. She had been able to work through the grief of her earlier miscarriage before discovering her true love in Tyler. She didn't feel the need to talk about the miscarriage with her husband, because it was something that happened with another man and was a wound that had already healed, a closed chapter in her life.

When I asked what would have made her feel more supported through her loss, Molly reiterated how alone she felt, even with Peter. "He was just scared and hiding in the background—always fifteen feet away," she teased, giggling now, "but behind the couch."

She is resolute about the importance of having doulas present and available to talk to women and their partners about pregnancy loss—preceding, during, and following a potential loss. Doulas know how to clean things up and provide care with a keen awareness and attention to what's needed, she feels—but if not a doula, then some other medical professional who can offer mental health services.

Molly, like so many of us, never had that follow-up care.

"We're left hovering with this open-endedness," she said. "But we need that grounding, the closure."

The loneliness was by far the most challenging aspect of the miscarriage. Even when people did show up, it felt like more of a "Facebook thing," Molly said—hollow and unsatisfying. A friend reached out on social media, inviting her to call, any time—but as badly as she wanted connection, Molly couldn't bring herself to reach out. She hadn't spoken with the woman in years and lacked the assertiveness to dial her number.

"I needed other people to come to me and show up."

I wondered aloud how we might better connect with others suffering from miscarriage. Whose responsibility is it? First, we have to know it's even happening to someone.

Molly circled back to the importance of bearing witness and the courage to share one's story. Opening up to share presents both a personal challenge and a broader public-health issue. For starters, people—physicians, doulas, friends, employers, partners—would need to listen and be prepared to act in service and with compassion.

"We heal through sharing our feelings and our stories. Space needs to be given to what is being felt, and that it's *allowed* to be named and felt and seen," Molly explained. "That's kind of all we need to get in touch with our own capacity to heal ourselves."

She also said she saw an opportunity in loss for connection as well as self-growth: "When we know how to share our stories and give them voice, it's a liberating tie that binds us to others and makes us more in touch with our own spirit and purpose."

Molly has seen a strength and resilience in herself and in her patients alike.

"This is a door that you're looking through," she offered, imagining a conversation with someone who recently experienced loss. "It's a good door, and I'm sorry it's so hard, but you're stronger and wiser now." Molly smiled at me. "You'll have so much more to offer this world, so much more appreciation for life."

With a caveat: be patient and kind to yourself. And please, Molly implored, break the silence.

CHAPTER 2

Desiree

"Feel what we feel and let it heal!"

WHAT FIRST STRUCK ME ABOUT DESIREE was her impeccably manicured yet effortless look. She stood tall and lithe, with bright, friendly eyes, glowing ivory skin, and a firmly rooted stance.

We met at a confidence-building workshop for mothers and daughters that I'd cohosted in Berkeley. She'd driven from Sacramento the night before with her two daughters, aged eleven and thirteen. She strode over to me with a disarming grin and outstretched hand. It was immediately clear to me that this woman already had a high degree of confidence. What she was there for was to connect with her daughters on a deeper level and support them in learning how to be strong and self-assured.

I was not surprised to learn that Desiree, forty-six, was a talent development coach and author who offered tough-love business consulting and what she called "inspiration for greatness." Even her darkest perspectives on miscarriage had an uplifting sense of hope and compassion. She was one of the first women to reach out to me when I announced my project.

Desiree legally separated from her husband, John, in 2017 and was in the process of divorce when we met on Zoom. When they married in 2003, family planning wasn't on her radar. While John was eager to become a father, she was reluctant, unsure of what it would mean for her career. Yet, true to her coaching nature, she was open to the possibility of kids and what might emerge. She had just turned thirty, and she and John were both fine with letting life unfold for them.

When she became pregnant later that year, Desiree and John were overcome with joy. They told close friends and relatives right away, and started thinking about what it would mean to grow their family. The Ob/Gyn confirmed the pregnancy around the eight-week mark, and they went in for their first prenatal visit at ten weeks. They couldn't wait to see the baby's heartbeat.

A nurse greeted them for the ultrasound. Desiree shared their excitement with her as John made jokes in his usual, chummy way of connecting with strangers. Desiree remembers the cold gel on her tummy, then looking over and beholding the wondrous grayscale of her baby.

Suddenly, the nurse stopped chatting with John and the room fell silent. She just needed a minute to focus, she told them. As she moved the wand around Desiree's belly the couple gazed at the monitor, in awe of the budding life inside her.

The nurse set aside the wand and lay a sheet over Desiree's midsection.

"What I think we have here is something called fetal demise." The nurse explained that she was unable to detect a heartbeat. "Now, because there's a possibility that I might be wrong, it's important that I get a physician to take a look as well."

The doctor confirmed their fears. No heartbeat. No baby. No laughter, which only moments ago had filled the room.

Desiree lay there stunned.

Her voice cracked as she tried to swallow back the tears. "All I could think was, *I broke my baby*," she shared with me on our video call, her cheeks wet and flushed. "*There's something wrong with me.*"

She recalled someone who had chided her earlier in the pregnancy, "Don't skip up those steps, you're pregnant!" as she playfully strode up a set of stairs. The guilty reel played over and over in her head.

"But what did I do wrong?" she wondered aloud to me, sniffling.

Breaking the silence in the exam room, the doctor shared that he and his wife had been a bit further along in their pregnancy when this same thing had happened to them. He, too, had struggled with the loss. He asked them to consider for a moment what it took to create a life form.

As Desiree relayed the doctor's words to me, her entire body perked up. She spoke with bravado, as if she were delivering a key-note speech.

"If you can imagine it," she began, "you have this complex DNA that needs to match up. Picture it like a progressive growth, where the first part of the DNA has to lock in, then the second, and the third, and so on. What happened with your pregnancy was that part one locked in, part two locked in, but somewhere down the line, a part couldn't lock in because something was a little off, so the process stopped and everything got broken down."

"When the time is right," he had assured them, "the process will start over for you."

Desiree paused and I suddenly felt that she wasn't just speaking about her own experience, she was speaking directly to me. *Would there ever be a right time for me?*

"There's nothing you could have done differently," she said, repeating her doctor's soothing words for me.

He had recognized Desiree's fears and immediately laid them to rest. She was relieved to know that she wasn't alone, or to blame for the loss.

When the doctor recommended a dilation and curettage (D&C), Desiree looked up, biting her lip. "I don't think I can do that." She didn't believe there was anything wrong with the surgical procedure, it just didn't feel right for her at the time. It felt like an admission that the baby was actually gone. "What are the other options?" she asked.

"Okay," he said, shifting his weight. "You're at a stage where you're far enough along that I have some concerns about you trying to wait this out, but you're not quite so far along that the complications would lead me to think that you wouldn't make it through. There's a risk either way."

He paused to make sure Desiree understood the risk that she might not pass the fetal tissue naturally. She nodded.

"Here's what I'll do," he offered. "I'd like to invite you back here in a week, and we'll check for the heartbeat again."

Desiree let out a sigh, relaxing her jaw.

"I want you to understand, though, that when you come back, we are not likely to hear anything."

Desiree nodded slowly, her eyes welled and fixed on the doctor.

"I think it'll help make this decision a little easier and give you some more time to be sure that this is a case of fetal demise." He looked from Desiree to John, then back to Desiree.

Desiree knew she couldn't terminate the pregnancy in her current emotional state. They thanked the doctor for the additional time and made their way home.

I asked Desiree what that waiting period was like for her.

"I spent the majority of the week in shock," she confided, her eyes still searching for the right word. "I think that's really what it was. Having just the tiniest sliver of hope." She lifted her hand, squinted through the tiny space she had created between her thumb and index finger, her mouth scrunched up toward her nose, and she sighed. "Yet being very realistic about the information we'd been given."

The time allowed her to digest the news and replay the conversations she'd had with the doctor and nurses. She thought about the baby and the beautiful images from the ultrasound.

She and John broke the tragic news to their friends and family and a neighbor across the street. As Desiree opened up, it seemed like everyone had a story to share—"Oh, I had a miscarriage" or "I remember when so-and-so had one."

Desiree found it disconcerting that women are congratulated for becoming pregnant. While she wouldn't expect anyone to say, "Hey, heads up, you might not make it to full term," or "Your body might decide that something won't lock in, and you'll lose the pregnancy," the high rates of miscarriage do suggest that many of those oft-congratulated pregnancies do not end successfully. So why, she wondered, haven't we normalized the dialogue around potential loss?

"It's like parenting," she said, craning her slender neck outward. "People try to tell you it's hard, but you can't hear it. There's the self-blame, the isolation—it's just a part of the human experience. But I had no idea how many people would say that they had gone through it themselves."

I wondered how that affected her at the time. Did it give her strength, as it had for me?

"At first it just made me think, *Am I around a bunch of people who happen to be the exception? Is this the norm?*"

When she returned to the doctor and received the final confirmation that her baby was gone, those stories provided much-needed comfort. By the end of the week, she understood that pregnancy loss was surprisingly common. Along with her doctor's initial explanation of miscarriage—stripped of shame, blame, or judgment, and rooted in tangible science—Desiree began to warm up to the idea of trying again to conceive. Not right away, but eventually.

She shook her head as she remarked how differently John processed the loss. "He'll go for the humor as soon as it's available to him. Of course, it wasn't available that first or second day." She cocked her head to the side and gasped. "Not that he'd ever make jokes about the miscarriage itself! It was just a redirection strategy." Focusing on other things, like work, was his way of coping.

John's mother lived nearby and was a support for them both. Of the four children she'd birthed, she'd lost one to Sudden Infant Death Syndrome (SIDS) and another as an adult. Having lived through the extreme ups and downs of birth and loss, she was a well of strength for Desiree.

"Giving me access to his parents and letting his mom comfort me at a time when he was also seeking comfort was incredibly generous of him," she told me, her eyes glistening.

John's mother accompanied her to the doctor for the follow-up visit, allowing John to get back to work with the confidence that Desiree was with someone he trusted. Once they had listened for the heart that Desiree had known—at least intellectually—had stopped beating, she was able to accept the miscarriage. Now she felt empowered to wait it out, to free herself physically from the loss, and continue moving through her grief. It took another week for the fetal tissue to pass naturally.

Given the circumstances, Desiree can't imagine having had a better medical-care experience.

"I made sure the whole time I was in that healthcare system that I stayed with him as my doctor," she said, her head tilted slightly upward and nodding. He went on to oversee the birth of her first daughter.

"When I got pregnant again, he understood. Every visit—every *successful* visit—he was celebrating in the same way we were."

I was curious to hear such a confident mother's advice for women experiencing pregnancy loss—but when I asked, Desiree at first claimed to have nothing to offer. I furrowed my brow, studying her relaxed expression, and waited for her voice to fill the space.

"What I *do* know is that my heart stayed open throughout that journey, and keeping my heart open was probably the most important thing I could do." Her tone was clear and steady as she leaned toward me. "But I'm not going to suggest that this would work for everybody. Sometimes we have to shell up before we can open again."

Desiree wondered aloud how the experience of sharing her miscarriage story back in 2003 would have compared with having that experience today, in our culture of instant and condensed connection via social media. If she posted, for instance, "I'm sad that this happened to me today," she might garner some hearts or teary-faced emojis, some well wishes and condolences, many of them impersonal-sounding though well-intentioned. But she doubted such responses would have as much impact as sharing directly with someone. That nuanced difference, she argued, allowed an opening for people not only to offer their comfort and care but also to share their own stories.

"There's something about the back-and-forth," she said, her upper body swaying side to side, "the dialogue, that's different from just a flat, 'Let me put it out there so you know you're not alone.' There's something about the exchange and the connection that we're able to make with one another."

Desiree's experience gelled with Molly's articulation of bearing witness, only with more specificity about the nature of the witnessing and sharing. Desiree believed it was the intimacy of in-person conversation that helped her through her experience. It wasn't about normalizing miscarriage itself; rather, it was about normalizing the *dialogue around* miscarriage, as well as other taboo subjects that touch our lives.

"We don't have to believe in suffering," she said with a lift in her voice. "We don't have to say, 'Oh, I'm sorry,' or 'I wish I could undo it for you'"—she paused and slowed her words—"but to say, 'I'm standing strong alongside you, and you're not alone.'"

While she knows she can't take away the pain and suffering, she also knows that people shouldn't have to endure it alone.

"We're just going to feel what we feel and let it heal!" she exclaimed with a palpable energy.

Desiree's words echoed in my mind like a rallying cheer through a stadium, reaffirming my dedication to this project. Nobody wanted to be a member of this club. Together, though, we could get through it. Together, with honest dialogue about our experiences of loss—and resilience.

CHAPTER 3

Ashley

"You don't have to be Wonder Woman."

ASHLEY APPEARED ON MY LAPTOP SCREEN made up for a cover shoot with cherry-red lips, rouged cheeks, smoky blue eyeliner, and thick mascara. When she reached for a loose strand of hair—which she failed to find, as they were all neatly gathered in the thick blond ponytail perched at the crown of her head—I noticed a freshly manicured porcelain hand, her nails a sleek gray.

As we introduced ourselves, she shifted in her seat, avoiding the camera, then looked at me with big doe eyes. She was nervous; she said she hoped it wouldn't be too much for me to hear her story.

She wiped tears from her face and told me about losing her parents: her father was killed by a home invader when she was seven, then her mother became wrapped up in an abusive relationship that rendered her unavailable as a parent.

The experience of growing up in an abusive home had left Ashley, now thirty, uninterested in having kids of her own. "Never really experiencing that solid family unit, I thought, *If this is what a relationship looks like, then I want nothing to do with it,*" she explained.

Although she lacked a father figure and wished for a better model for a husband than she'd seen with her mother, Ashley was surprisingly unafraid of romantic love or commitment. She eloped at twenty with David, a boyfriend she'd met as a teenager, and a few years into their marriage, she began wondering if she and David could create a different kind of family from the troubled one she'd known as a child. She confided those doubts to her maternal grandmother, an ordained minister.

"Sweetheart," Grammy told her, "don't let the past define your future."

David was fully on board. Of course they could forge a different path, and for him that absolutely meant having kids.

With her grandmother's support, Ashley soon embraced the idea of motherhood with open arms—and she got pregnant right away.

Shortly after the first prenatal visit, at eight weeks, she and David went to a friend's birthday dinner. They came home late, happy, and sated, and fell asleep. In the middle of the night, Ashley woke up cramping and instantly regretted that second piece of cake. When she flicked on the bathroom light, she was shocked to see blood pooling on the floor. She panicked and called for David. Observing the crimson mess, they knew something was wrong and immediately drove to the hospital.

Ashley wasn't conscious of any pain, only the sensation of cramping. In the car, she called her mother, who shot out of bed to meet them at the hospital. She also rang one of her friends who had lost her first pregnancy. She was the only woman besides her mother that Ashley knew of who'd had a miscarriage. She wasn't sure what her friend could tell her, she just wanted to hear her voice. She ended up leaving a message.

When they got to the hospital, a nurse quickly showed them to a room, but everything else played out in slow motion. Ashley went through hours of testing, then waiting, then more tests and waiting.

Everyone seemed to know what was happening—the doctors and nurses, Ashley's mother, David, even Ashley herself. But the staff wouldn't say it was a miscarriage until they ran through all the tests. Ashley didn't need them to say anything; all she needed was David's arms around her.

Before that night, Ashley didn't know that ultrasounds could be performed vaginally. She distinctly remembered the coldness of the wand, as well as the technician, who had a chilly nonchalance about him.

"Here he was, invading my body in a way nobody else would," she told me. "Such an intimate, emotional experience. It was traumatic, yet he was acting like he didn't even care." She was bleeding so heavily that she had to swap out her soiled hospital gowns for fresh ones several times.

Hours later, one of the nurses spoke with the couple. Her tone was different from the ultrasound technician's—softer, sympathetic. To Ashley's relief, she didn't sugarcoat the news. Shortly afterward, the family doctor showed similar warmth and steadiness.

Soon, they were told they could go home. When the staff went to remove Ashley's IV, she was suddenly struck with terror, confused about the tube in her arm. As her heart rate plummeted and her vision became spotty with faintness, the nurse instructed her to lie back down.

Once Ashley had stabilized, the nurse walked her and David out.

"I can tell you two really love each other," she told them. "You're going to get through this together. You're young, and you have a lot of life ahead of you. There will be many more opportunities."

As soon as Ashley and David got in the car, they broke down sobbing.

Recounting this moment, Ashley apologized to me for crying as she dabbed at her eyes. I understood that feeling of having to hold it together till I could be untamed in my emotions in private. I hadn't wanted anyone to see my pain or sadness, to have to hold the ten-ton weight I imagined myself to be, after my miscarriage.

In the sanctuary of their hatchback, Ashley spent the next half hour with her head buried in her husband's chest. She felt like a part of their lives had been taken away from them. Maybe it was harder because they hadn't initially wanted a family, and then had intentionally chosen that path for themselves. Could it really be gone, just like that? She felt herself losing control—assuming she'd ever had it in the first place. The world was crumbling around her, and all she could do was sit in a parking lot and cry.

Yet Ashley knew David was there with her, feeling those same emotions. Even if he couldn't change what had happened, even if they couldn't comfort one another in this moment, at least there was something, someone, to hold on to.

As the days wore on, a numbness settled over Ashley, which gave way to a darkness she had never felt before or since. She began to question if she had done something wrong. Although her doctor, family, and friends all assured her it wasn't her fault, the words didn't quite sink into her heart. She felt frustrated, ashamed to be a woman who couldn't carry a child to term. She told herself she wasn't enough of a woman, or even enough of a human. She considered herself a complete failure.

Even when the suicidal thoughts began, Ashley didn't want to seem needy or burden anyone by divulging them. She wanted nothing more than to move beyond her loss and get on with her life.

She felt isolated and removed, frozen in her darkness.

Yet she wasn't entirely alone. When the cramping continued well after the bleeding subsided, David showed his support by fetching her heating pads for her back and making sure she was reasonably comfortable. The pain was at times excruciating, but eventually it stopped.

To her complete surprise, Ashley had a period just weeks after the miscarriage. She was entering a classroom on campus when she felt a rush of blood exit her body. When she got to the bathroom to assess, she was unprepared for the heavy flow. She took refuge outside by a rock wall that mostly covered her stained jeans while she waited for her husband to bring her a change of clothes and drive her home.

She wished she could have laughed it off, but the humiliation was too great. She had thought she was finally in the clear, at least physically, but now the menstrual cramping she was experiencing was reminding her of the emotional pain of her loss. Just as she was regaining control of her life and getting back into the swing of things, here she was, missing class again, helpless and embarrassed, pulling her husband out of work to care for her.

And even in this numb limbo, she still had her usual responsibilities to juggle. "I had to create a second self and wear this mask at work and school."

She wasn't always able to keep up the facade. Right after the loss, when she was having an especially difficult morning, she messaged one of her professors to say she couldn't make it to class. The professor's response still made her choke up.

She told Ashley she was sorry it happened. She'd had a miscarriage, too, when she was younger. She encouraged Ashley to take all the time she needed.

Postpartum depression (PPD) is common among women who have miscarried, not unlike women who've given birth at full term. As the body goes through dramatic changes to accommodate the postpartum phase—be it breastfeeding or rebuilding the uterine walls— the plummeting and surging of various hormones can cause massive shifts in emotions and regulation. For many women, this results in mild to severe depression that typically lasts up to six weeks.[4]

Ashley experienced severe postpartum symptoms for the better part of a week.

"I felt like I should just drive off a cliff: I couldn't do anything right. I couldn't even do basic woman things right!" she recalled, tears streaming down her rosy cheeks.

While most women experience the "baby blues," approximately 15 percent of women develop clinical postpartum depression[5,6]. However, it is the exception rather than the rule for family doctors or Ob/Gyn staff to inform patients about the warning signs and risks of PPD. This is especially true for women who have miscarried. It's unusual for staff to offer them any resources before they leave the site of care. And even when what little support there is gets offered, many women feel too ashamed or selfish to accept it.

Ashley felt motivated to share her story to help women understand that they're not alone. Though it may be difficult to ask for help, she insisted that support is out there. Her voice, which had wavered throughout our conversation, was at once clear and confident as she said, "I wouldn't want any other woman in my situation to have those feelings." She looking upward, willing her tears to stay at bay. But there was no stopping them as she paused to reflect on that dark chapter of her life.

I told Ashley how brave she was to share her story. Her lips slowly curled into a smile as she thanked me and dried her eyes.

Shortly after the miscarriage, Ashley's grandmother sent her a note confiding that she, too, had lost a pregnancy and had found healing through memorializing the loss. She recommended that Ashley name the baby and find some way to honor it. So she and David chose a name and had a small memorial service, just the two of them, with flowers and a proper good-bye by a creek near their home.

A handful of Ashley's closest friends also reached out to comfort her. They were mindful of giving her and David space to grieve, so they told her that they would just drop off dinners. They didn't ask, they simply let them know they would do it. So as not to intrude, they delivered the meals on the doorstep, rang the bell, and took off. It was a relief not to have to make small talk but still feel her friends' support.

Others were less sensitive to her tender state. One friend made a comment that left a particularly bad taste in her mouth: "Something was probably wrong with the baby, Ashley. It was all for the better."

Except it wasn't all better. Nothing was better. While her doctor had explained to her that miscarriage was often the body's means of self-terminating a complicated pregnancy, it wasn't what she wanted to hear from a friend.

"I didn't want anyone to find silver linings for me," she explained. "It felt shallow and inauthentic and insulting. I just needed people to recognize the pain and be there."

For loved ones to show up and acknowledge the loss without putting a positive spin on it is what so many women say they need and so rarely get. As a friend or family member unfamiliar with this kind of loss—or any loss, for that matter—it can be challenging to be around people in grief and mourning. Many find it frustrating and defeating to be in grief's company, unable to do or say anything to lift the spirits of the bereaved. Understandably, many of us fumble and end up further alienating them. Ashley didn't begrudge her friends who, despite their best intentions, made her feel worse and even further disconnected.

She did, however, feel that the medical community could and should have done more to help. Nobody bothered to follow up with her, save for a routine pap smear she was told to go in for weeks after her miscarriage. Nobody warned her about the grieving process, let alone the possibility of postpartum depression. She was never offered an opportunity to talk with a social worker or therapist who might have been able to help her through the depression.

"My friends tried so hard to be the professionals, but they weren't," she explained.

I asked Ashley if she could articulate a better version of the aftercare she wished other women experiencing pregnancy loss would receive. She barely skipped a beat before responding.

What if, she proposed, instead of sending women home and

scratching them off their patient lists, hospitals and clinics took proactive steps to help us understand how to work through the loss and manage grief's complex emotions? For instance, they could distribute pamphlets about support groups or send in a roaming social worker to talk with women and couples about the transition and what to expect. Staff could let patients know that someone would call to check in on their physical and mental well-being. They could even invite patients to schedule a follow-up appointment on their own to talk through any issues or concerns.

Ashley feels frustrated that no one ever mentioned miscarriage in any of her routine gynecological exams or even prenatal visits. Maybe if she had understood how common it was and what kind of emotional impact it could have, she wouldn't have felt so alienated. She might have coped better knowing in advance what to expect and how to handle the pitfalls. She might've even been able to ask for help without feeling ashamed.

Ashley knows there were some resources online at the time; in fact, doing that research was part of David's grieving and sense-making process. But it didn't resonate for her. She didn't feel like wading through it all. If a professional or someone she knew who'd had a miscarriage had been able to say to her, "check out this website," "read this," or "listen to this podcast," however, maybe she would have. She certainly wanted that connection with other women who'd been through it, but she felt too dark and depressed to make the effort on her own. She just wished she had been better prepared before it all happened.

Ashley wonders if we could increase awareness by making it part of sex education. That way, girls and boys would understand that pregnancies don't always have a Hollywood ending. We wouldn't judge or assign blame or failure to a woman or her body. We wouldn't assume that all pregnancies lead to successful births and happy families.

After the baby's due date had come and gone—an event accompanied by many heavy emotions—Ashley was ready to try again, this time without the expectation of guaranteed success. Once she was pregnant, she lived in constant fear of losing the baby, even after they'd reached the major milestones: at nine weeks, when they lost their first baby; at twelve weeks, when most vital organs are formed; and at twenty-four weeks, when a fetus is understood to be viable outside the womb.

With each new hurdle, she and David breathed a little sigh of relief. But there was always that thought in the back of her mind, *What if something happens?*

"There was nothing I could have done with the first one, and I was so afraid of that happening again," she said, swallowing back tears.

Ashley's subsequent pregnancies gave her two healthy children, now seven and four and a half. They decided to announce both pregnancies after twenty-four weeks.

As she reflected on her experience, Ashley was struck by the depth of her emotion, both positive and negative. On the one hand, she discovered she has the capacity for an all-consuming love for her unborn child; on the other, a level of depression and shame she never knew was possible.

Over time, Ashley recognized how she'd internalized the negative emotions. She worked to communicate better about those pain points, bringing others into the conversation earlier and in a way where she felt safe before things got too dark and she lost her compass. She was determined to never again let herself suffer alone.

She wishes now that she hadn't felt so much pressure to move on from her loss.

"The world expects people to just get up and keep going," she told me. "And because so many women keep these experiences hidden, we never see that others *are* taking the time they need to process." Ashley certainly wishes she had. "You don't have to be Wonder Woman," she urged. "Take the time."

She said that now that her children are older, she's been wondering if and how to tell them about the first pregnancy, the child who would've been their older sibling. She can't imagine ever forgetting that child or the grief its loss still causes her.

"The pain doesn't go away, you just learn how to manage it."

Ashley patted the corners of her eyes, makeup fully intact, and flashed me a big smile. After we said our good-byes, I stopped the recording and reached for a box of tissues, wishing I could go back in time and hold her in my arms.

CHAPTER 4

Suzy

"No baby, no client."

"IF SOMEONE HANDED ME ANOTHER BABY, I'd be drowning in babies. I wouldn't even know what to do. We're potty training all day, every day."

I imagined a small army of redheaded children clambering up their mother's wide frame and into her carrot top of corkscrew curls.

Suzy, a thirty-nine-year-old engineering scientist in Bellevue, Illinois, and her ginger-bearded husband, Will, both come from large families. They always wanted one for themselves too, at least three kids. They even talked about a fourth, but given the current circus—"I think we're good," Suzy said.

When they first got married and still lived in New Jersey, Suzy spoke to her Ob/Gyn about family planning. Then thirty-three, she was concerned about risk factors for older women and wanted the facts without the candy coating. Dr. Smolinsky reassured her with a flick of her hand, "You're fine! You're young, strong, and healthy. I see you having many babies."

Soon enough, Suzy was pregnant with their honeymoon baby, William Junior.

Dr. Smolinsky worked out of a small office and outsourced

routine procedures like sonograms to larger facilities, where Suzy didn't always hear her OB's level of optimism. Early in her second trimester, one doctor pressured Suzy to get an amniocentesis—still considered the gold standard for prenatal genetic diagnostic testing despite its high cost and invasive nature, and the fact that it increases risk of miscarriage. While alternative methods are now considered safer and more effective, the test was traditionally recommended to women thirty-five and older.

Suzy refused.

"We don't want anything *like* that!" she told the doctor who was pushing for it. "We're fully committed to having this baby, regard-less." Suzy knew that standard blood work for women her age, then thirty-four, already included basic genetic testing.

The doctor initially persisted, but eventually backed down. Suzy suspected that he was more concerned about his liability than her well-being.

"I get it," she explained to me over Zoom, "people will sue you as a doctor. But there's a more delicate way to communicate the risks for older women."

Shortly after the visit, the doctor called with the results of the basic testing. He told her the fetus had tested positive for Down Syndrome, citing a mere one in ninety-six chance of her child having the disorder. A genetic counselor would call her to follow up with more information.

Suzy hung up and broke into tears. She relayed the news to Will, then called Dr. Smolinsky's office. A nurse assured her there was nothing to worry about: "Suzy, please. Don't even let your mind go there." Suzy and Will were having a boy and, as the nurse explained, those tests sometimes show misleading levels for males. The results were inconclusive, and follow-up tests would soon rule anything out.

The second round of testing came back completely normal. Suzy's blood boiled thinking how irresponsible her doctor had been, making a huge fuss over nothing.

"As a first-time parent, you don't know what's going on. You don't know what to expect, and you're at the mercy of your doctor's words," she told me, throwing her arms in the air.

Suzy wasn't just disappointed—she was furious that the doctor hadn't given her the underlying data associated with those results. She was a scientist, after all. She understood data. And regardless of their familiarity with numbers, she argued, patients deserve both the detailed results and the credit for being able to make sense of them. No one should have to hear that they've "tested positive" for inconclusive results, especially those based on a 1 percent probability.

William wasn't born with Down Syndrome.

"We have a beautiful boy who's verbal and fantastic. There are challenges, sure, but he's our wonderful William! I mean, Down Syndrome?" she asked, her voice climbing a full register. "It's just Down Syndrome! We could've managed that. But there's a better way to communicate risk, and they really dropped the ball on that."

Not long after William Jr. was able to walk, Dr. Smolinsky helped deliver baby Audrey. Suzy had just finished maternity leave when the family moved to the Midwest for Will Sr.'s work.

The couple was excited to grow the family, and Suzy was soon pregnant for the third time. Just days before her eight-week prenatal appointment, she started bleeding and knew something was wrong. She called her new OB, who told her to come into the office.

After completing the blood work, Suzy asked when she would see her doctor. "Oh, that won't be necessary," a nurse explained, waving her off.

Suzy relayed this to me with a sassy "talk to the hand" gesture. Underneath her joking facade, I saw a burning frustration.

The following day, a nurse called Suzy to request that she come in for more blood work. The matter was somewhat complicated by the fact that Suzy has type O-negative blood and her husband does not. She was instructed to get a RhoGAM shot—something generally recommended after a miscarriage as a precaution against a situation called Rh incompatibility, which can affect future pregnancies— right away.

Without explicitly acknowledging it, the nurse had insinuated that Suzy had lost the pregnancy. But Suzy needed to hear it more bluntly; hope still flickered in her heart.

The OB's office didn't have the shot on hand, so staff sent her to the hospital. To Suzy's shock, a roaming nurse, after glancing at her chart, offered her condolences for her loss. She reassured Suzy it was just something that happens, and not to take it personally.

That's when the grief hit. Suzy burst into tears as soon as she left the hospital, a visceral sadness flooding her entire bloodstream.

"It's so sudden!" she recalled. "You take it all the way to the baby, and you're thinking names and color schemes . . . But, in reality, it's like"—her voice dropped to a whisper—"okay, no, this isn't happening."

A nurse called a few days later and told Suzy to return for more blood work. By then, staff had canceled her original appointment, but she still hadn't spoken with her doctor. When she asked when that would happen, a different nurse explained it wouldn't be necessary.

"You become second class!" Suzy fumed, shaking her head. "They're in the business of babies, so when you're not having a baby, you're no longer a client!"

After her lab work, someone called to report that her levels of the pregnancy hormone HCG had dropped to nearly zero, so she wouldn't need to come back for further testing. Suzy politely thanked the nurse and inquired about follow-up care.

"What follow-up care?" the woman replied.

Suzy was floored. She still had questions about her health and how to proceed. She wanted to know when it would be safe to start trying again. Should she wait? What would the healing process be like? Was there anything she should know?

The nurse told her that a miscarriage typically means that something went wrong, and Suzy should wait until she got her period before trying again to conceive. Then she hung up.

Suzy bled for nearly two weeks and not once saw or even spoke with a doctor. The bill for the RhoGAM shot ($500) came several months later—a final, gut-punch reminder of the loss.

Outraged by her OB's lack of support, Suzy found a new Ob/Gyn practice; it was farther from her home, but the difference in care was worth the extra drive. It was a larger practice with doctors in rotation, but the staff was kind and respectful and the care was continuous. They understood about the recent miscarriage, and were sensitive to it without tiptoeing around it.

I asked Suzy how she and Will coped with the loss.

"We were in shock," she said softly. "It sucks, but there's nothing you can do about it."

She wondered if she could have done anything differently, though she knew better than to blame herself. She browsed online for support but didn't find much that spoke to her. She figures now that she could have reached out to Cigna, her insurer, for additional information, but who had time for that? She was juggling two toddlers and a full-time job.

Suzy and Will didn't tell anyone at first. They hadn't even told people they were pregnant. They usually waited until twelve weeks. Suzy's parents came out for Christmas that year, so they told them along with Will's mother.

"We wanted to keep it private, because we didn't know how to process it," Suzy explained. "We didn't know how to grieve about it." She fiddled with the arm of her chair, then let out a big sigh. "I didn't want to tell anybody 'cause I didn't want them to be like, 'Are you okay?'"

She winced and quickly shook her head, as if she were flicking away the discomfort of the experience.

"I just wanted to be done with it."

Eventually, the couple did start talking about it. One of Will's close friends at work, Sarah, had a miscarriage at twelve weeks. Will shared with her that they'd been through something similar, offered his support, and suggested that she talk to Suzy.

Suzy was happy to connect and found that Sarah—like Suzy, Desiree, and so many others—was completely unaware that she knew anyone who'd miscarried until she opened up about her loss. Suddenly, the floodgates also opened.

"Nobody talks about it until it happens," Suzy said, describing what was becoming an emphatic theme. "Then suddenly everyone they know is gasping, 'Me too! Me too!'"

Suzy saw an inherent danger and absurdity in women and doctors continuing to avoid the subject, particularly for the growing number of women choosing to have children later in life. As the risks for miscarriage increase with maternal age, this is an issue that's affecting even more women and families today than it has in the past. Yet, to Suzy's vexation, we still aren't talking about it.

"Make it a conversation because, right now, there is no conversation," she urged with a thrust of her neck.

Having just moved to the Midwest, away from most of her friends and family, it had been hard for Suzy to imagine those conversations. "I mean, everyone's very pleasant," she said slowly, choosing her words. *Let's face it,* her ensuing sigh told me, *miscarriage isn't exactly a pleasant topic to bring up with your neighbors and colleagues.*

The relative isolation did, however, bring Suzy and Will closer together as a couple. They also found that opening up to friends and family who'd experienced miscarriage allowed them to feel less helpless in their own situation and more helpful to others. But it took time to get there. They each needed to process on their own before they were ready to explore the subject together and then with others.

Six weeks after miscarrying, Suzy learned she was pregnant again. Instantly, an anxious cloud loomed over her. She constantly questioned the viability. Adding to that uncertainty, she actually lost weight during her pregnancy, which worried her; in her past pregnancies, she had gained an average of sixty-five pounds. This time, she had lost fifteen.

"Honestly, I thought I had leukemia!" Her emerald eyes darted back and forth, channeling the anxiety she felt at the time.

The doctors, however, reassured her everything was fine: "This baby just carries differently," they told her.

Laughing, Suzy relayed their efforts to cheer her up: "It's your skinny baby time! Enjoy it!"

By far, little Trixie was her easiest pregnancy. None of the excruciating pain of kidney stones that she had had with the other kids. Perfectly uneventful.

Yet the fear of losing the baby never went away.

She was out one day mowing the lawn, feeling great. Then a panic seized her. She was the most petitely pregnant she'd ever been—fragile, even. She should be taking it easy, not doing yard work! But how could she know what was safe anymore? How could she trust her body?

"You're never in a comfortable place," she said. "Our friends in Jersey lost at twenty-one weeks. You hear horror stories! The whole time it's just incredibly delicate."

Generally, when women are further along in their pregnancy, and even postpartum, there are a whole slew of checklists, with all sorts of health professionals asking questions and checking in. A nurse sits down with a woman in her third trimester to make sure she's not experiencing adverse symptoms. Yet this is far from standard practice for women who miscarry. Follow-up care is essentially nonexistent.

"Back of the bus!" Suzy yelled. "They don't care. No baby, no client! As if there's nothing they can do for you." She flung her arms up in the air. "But there should be!" Her voice leveled off. "That step is obviously missing. They should at least do some screening to make sure you don't need any other care, or"—her voice rose again—"or a conversation! Come on!"

Suzy never got that conversation. She never heard, "If you have questions, call this number or go to this website." No, "Here are some people who went through exactly what you went through." No, "Here's all the questions you might have, with all the answers you need to know."

The extent of Suzy's follow-up care was someone telling her to come in for another lab so they could eventually scratch her off their list the minute her HCG levels bottomed out.

"It's the most impersonal thing we ever went through with the medical field," Suzy said flatly.

She wanted to believe that if she had had her miscarriage under the care of Dr. Smolinsky, back in New Jersey, it would have gone differently. But she wasn't so sure. Not one of the miscarriage mothers she had spoken with received any aftercare.

Clearly, there is a need for follow-up. Mental health issues often include anxiety, grief, and depression. With the physical symptoms, such as cramping and blood loss, women typically don't know if their experience is normal because nobody's ever discussed what to expect.

"It's an intimate thing women physically endure," Suzy explained. "My husband's awesome, but he didn't go through it. He totally feels for it emotionally, but physically? My hormones are different, everything's different!"

Like Ashley, Suzy wished more information had been offered to her up front to help her manage her expectations and feel better prepared for a potential loss. It would have been helpful to be referred to a therapist early on—someone she could talk to about what she was going through—and to hear about common pregnancy challenges. And while there tended to be more communication with women who were further along in their pregnancies, even then, Suzy felt it was lacking.

"Just tell them everything!" she pleaded, her eyes growing wider. "I mean, they give you a pamphlet at your first prenatal visit with all sorts of information. But why doesn't it have *that* information?"

From Suzy's perspective, the medical community didn't get how to talk with women. She said that when she was pregnant with Audrey, she asked to schedule her remaining appointments at her first well visit, and the nurse wouldn't do it.

"Honey, no!" Suzy mocked the woman in a high-pitched tone. "You're not ready for that. It's still too early." If the nurse was trying for empathy, Suzy certainly wasn't feeling it.

In her view, there has to be a better way for providers to talk about the risk of pregnancy loss. "Maybe it's an insurance thing," she mused. "It's big business all around. But insurers and doctors need that other layer of therapy or counseling in there—'woman counseling,' whatever you want to call it!"

Infuriating as the experience was, it made Suzy recognize her own strength. She vividly remembers how devastating it felt to be alone and unsure about what was happening with her body, and how she realized early on that in order to get through her miscarriage, she would have to be her own advocate: do her own research and ask the tough questions herself. She couldn't just wait around anymore. Although it shouldn't be this way, her takeaway was that women must self-advocate and find support on their own.

Suzy's final words of advice?

"Take the time to really process the emotions. I wasn't ready at first. I wasn't ready to tell my parents or anyone really. It was easier to keep it between me and my husband. But when I started to hear stories of other people going through it, I knew it was time to share."

When Suzy's younger brothers started having children, she shared her tips and experiences with their wives, including what she'd learned from her miscarriage. "We need to keep the communication open and share what happened to us in the hopes that it will help others," she said.

Suzy's most encouraging words were infused with anger. As we ended our video call, I felt that anger reverberate through my body; my skin was flushed, my jaw tight. Lingering at my desk with this tension, I grew increasingly agitated until I cracked open my laptop and began to write. Suddenly, I understood how this anger could catalyze change—sparking the dialogue so many keep hush.

CHAPTER 5

Kari

"As a woman of color, I really expected more."

"I'M TELLING YOU BOYS, I'm going into labor," the woman said, huffing her way to the intake desk.

The paramedics, a pair of burly, clean-shaven men in their late-twenties, exchanged skeptical glances. The woman's ashen forearms, a splotchy constellation of purple lines and blackened circles, elucidated the nature of her visit to the Emergency Department. She looked too old to be pregnant, though they'd seen so often how abuse could age a person.

Kari, a clinical nurse specialist with a mocha complexion and smiling brown eyes, was making her rounds when she noticed the older Black woman. There was something about her. Kari needed to be by her side.

So, when she finished her lap around the ward, she went looking for her.

Kari found her lying on a gurney awaiting an ultrasound. The doctors wanted to eliminate the possibility of pregnancy and move on to more pressing patients.

Kari nodded at the technician setting up the monitor and went over to hold the woman's hand.

"Ma'am, I gotta use the restroom," the woman said, her breath growing heavier.

"Okay, well let's get you up," Kari said cheerily, offering her arm. "Nice and easy." The woman's forehead was damp with exertion. "Good. Deep breaths now."

When they made it to the bathroom, Kari helped pull down her pants—and the next thing she knew, the woman had given birth on the floor.

Kari stood there and let her squeeze her hand, squeeze the life out of it, while she helped her deliver a beautiful, almond-skinned, healthy girl.

"Sugar, I gotta tell you," the woman confessed, "I been using this whole pregnancy."

Kari took in the information with a clenched jaw, forcing back tears. "It'll be okay," she told her.

Later that day, Kari went up to the neonatal intensive care unit (NICU) and tracked down the woman's baby in an incubator. The woman had already checked herself out, and it was obvious she wouldn't be returning. Kari cried as the little girl's chest rose and fell with each breath.

Some of the other nurses gathered around and, in hushed voices, asked what was wrong.

"It just doesn't seem fair for this child," she managed.

What she didn't say was that she'd recently suffered a miscarriage, and that she'd wanted that baby more than she'd been able to comprehend until this very moment. Her emotions were too raw to mention these things at work—or anywhere, for that matter, outside the safety of her marriage.

A part of Kari empathized with the woman who'd deserted her baby. She probably thought that, as an active drug user, she was doing the right thing. But where was God?

"The injustice of it all," Kari cried to me, gasping for breath between sobs. "She abandoned that baby in the hospital and I—I would have given anything . . ."

Kari, forty-five, was born into a strict religious family in Trinidad and spent most of her life in Maryland. She met her husband, Jon, a white man six years her senior, in the fall of 2011. He'd been married before and immediately recognized a kindred spirit and lifelong partner in Kari. He proposed eight months into their courtship, and they married the following spring.

Neither Kari nor Jon came into the marriage with children, but they'd always imagined becoming parents. As soon as they tied the knot, they started trying.

"It was a happy time," Kari reminisced with twinkling eyes. "We were newlyweds in a fresh relationship, just so excited about the prospect of getting pregnant." She sighed. "Even though we hadn't been together that long, we were so ready for it."

By October of that year, Kari had conceived. The night she tested positive, she and Jon cuddled on the sofa and made plans for a long weekend celebration in Monticello, Virginia. They buzzed with excitement as they looked at landmark inns and imagined their baby's features and personality.

Eight weeks into the pregnancy, during their special getaway, Kari noticed some spotting. She mentioned it to Jon, but assured him there was no cause for alarm. As a nurse, she'd seen her fair share of miscarriages and stillbirths, but she also knew that spotting was a common symptom of early pregnancies.

Kari's Ob/Gyn told her not to fret when she called, and scheduled her for her first prenatal visit and ultrasound that week. Kari trusted her doctor. She'd specifically sought out a practice with Black women doctors who could better serve patients like herself. She implicitly had more faith in her medical team than she did in the predominantly white men she tended to see elsewhere in the field—even in a city like Baltimore, where whites make up less than a third of the population.

Kari hadn't experienced any pregnancy symptoms like morning sickness or food cravings. This initially worried her, but she let go of any anxiety after her mother claimed she'd never had any symptoms when pregnant with both Kari and her sister.

While Kari didn't *feel* pregnant, she'd tested positive at home and missed three periods. Her cycle was irregular, however, so she hoped the ultrasound would reveal how far along she was.

On the eve of her ultrasound, Kari woke before dawn doubled over in pain. Jon was working nights, so she was on her own.

"I'd had cramps with my periods," Kari told me, "but, my gosh, never to this point." She shuddered with the memory.

Bleeding began by the time Jon got home in the morning. Kari knew the risk she faced if this were an ectopic pregnancy, so she asked Jon to drive her to the hospital.

"Oh, I'll never forget it." Kari laughed nervously as she recalled the experience. "The first doctor who talked to me was trying to keep me calm and reassure me that this didn't mean it was the end." She swallowed audibly. "But it was a pretty long wait . . . too long for someone in my condition."

Eventually, Kari received a transvaginal ultrasound. She bled profusely through the whole thing. The technician wouldn't tell her anything except that a doctor would be by soon.

Kari was shocked that in the nearly seven hours of dreadful waiting, not a single nurse came to help her. Nobody even offered her a menstrual pad for the bleeding. After several hours, Jon began wandering the halls of the ED, asking for a pad for his wife.

"People poked their heads in the room to ask about my pain level, but they never offered any pain medicine." Kari's usually sweet, low voice picked up some fire. "And that was the worst pain in my life!" She laughed to defuse the tension that was clearly rising inside her.

Hours after the ultrasound, a new doctor appeared.

"Okay, what's going on?" Kari asked him pointedly.

Jon stood by her side, eyes tired but hopeful, and caressed her hand.

"We were able to see the gestational sac," the doctor said curtly. "It was empty."

Kari burst into tears, her body bobbing like a buoy in the harbor. Jon squeezed her hand and listened intently as the doctor walked them through their options.

"You could have a D&C," the doctor started, "take the misoprostol pills, try the suppository . . ." His words faded as the deafening weight in Kari's chest, combined with the painful throbbing of her pelvis, drowned them out.

Kari didn't want a procedure. Her body was cramping and bleeding so much, she assumed it was already doing the heavy lifting. She opted for the least invasive route: the misoprostol.

Before she was discharged, a nurse came in to take her vitals.

"Belly out to there!" Kari described the woman, her arms outstretched. "I just broke down sobbing."

The woman ignored her crying, made some notes in her chart, and left the room.

"You know, where I've worked as a nurse, we go the extra step to make sure that women who miscarry don't have a visibly pregnant person caring for them." Kari shook her head, lips pursed. "Clearly, they never considered that with me."

She still has bitterness about it to this day.

"Listen, I'm an emergency room nurse, so I get that I wasn't a life-threatening case, I wasn't their highest priority"—her voice rose—"but nursing was not there. Knowing what nursing care should look like, that experience will never leave me. Insult to injury."

Kari spent the next few days weeping and sleeping or on the toilet passing the fetal tissue.

Jon, who'd taken some days off to be with her, grew concerned. He desperately wanted to cheer her up. Five years earlier, when his ex-wife had suffered a miscarriage, he wished he had been more sup-portive. They hadn't known the gender yet, but Jon had wanted a son so badly, he'd already thought of a name. The loss was in the back of their minds when he and Kari were trying to conceive, and here it was present with him again as he wondered how best to console his wife.

On the fourth day holed up in bed, not once having come down-stairs, let alone left the house, Kari's senses were suddenly awakened. The fatty, umami, brown-sugar aroma was unmistakable. She extri-cated herself from the tangle of blankets and heating pads, walked the few steps to the bedroom door, and stuck her head out into the hallway, where the smell of sizzling bacon reminded her she hadn't eaten anything in days.

Within minutes, she was fully dressed and feasting at the kitchen table.

"I doubt I would have managed to get out of that depression with-out him," Kari gushed. "He really wanted to make sure I got back to life."

Besides her husband, those closest to Kari did their best to be supportive, but their efforts, as is often the case with grief, fell short.

"My family tried," she explained. "I don't think they realized some of the things they said were more hurtful than helpful."

"Well, we just need to pray," her mother offered, but those com-ments ultimately eroded Kari's Christian faith. Kari felt the sting of judgment in her mother's suggestion to pray, or pray harder.

"I prayed nonstop during the whole pregnancy, and I still miscar-ried," Kari said. "My mom meant well but it still hurt. Like somehow my faith wasn't enough to keep me from miscarrying."

Her closest friends, all childless, made their best efforts to com-fort Kari, telling her the experience wasn't a big deal.

"You're still young," they said, "you can always try again."

"I can *kind* of see where they were coming from," Kari told me with a dubious lilt of her voice. "But their comments were still hurt-ful." She eked out a nervous chuckle.

While dispirited by the lack of support from her immediate circle, Kari was ravaged by her doctor's response. She'd explicitly sought out a woman of color to be her OB, expecting relatability and better care, but when she asked if there were any support groups she could join her doctor shrugged, confused as to why Kari would need a support group when the pregnancy hadn't been that far along.

This dismissiveness threw Kari off guard. She had expected more support from her people—and from a woman, no less. Why was the world so insensitive to her loss? Was she missing something?

"Their whole advertisement was about being a practice of women of color, so I figure they're here to help women of color," she told me. "This being Baltimore, there's plenty of us who need help."

The disappointment Kari felt stemmed from her presumption of a sisterhood amongst Black women. When her unspoken expectations of support went unmet, she experienced an even greater letdown than she would have from, say, a white male OB.

Such are the complexities of feminism and intersectionality.[7] Many of us from various ethnicities, classes, sexual orientations, etc. assume that people "like us" will be more compassionate to our plight, and then when those people show a stronger preference toward an identity that does not align with ours, we feel betrayed. What unites us superficially and experientially doesn't always deter-mine how we'll think or act. Alternatively, anything outside of what unites us may be seen as a perceived threat.

"I think we expect that we'll be there for each other," Kari said. "Black women support everyone, right? Sometimes to our detriment! So when we don't see that support from other Black women, it's deva-stating." She shook her head and grunted out a little laugh. "That OB's simple facial expression prevented me from getting the very help I now know I could have used."

This incident made Kari wonder if her husband's whiteness had something to do with her OB's reaction. But she chose not to pursue the race issue and never bothered looking elsewhere for support.

A few months later, Kari became pregnant again. She switched Ob/Gyn practices when she found out. While her new doctor wasn't Black, she was Indian, and Kari was still comforted and hopeful to be in the care of another woman of color.

Only a week passed between the day Kari tested positive at home and the day she had her first contractions of miscarriage, but it felt like a lifetime. With the first loss still fresh in her mind, she was on hyperalert. Every time she went to the bathroom, she looked for spotting. Any little twinge in her body threw her into worry—*Is that gas pain from the sandwich I just ate or is it happening again?* Her lack of symptoms now put her on edge. She downloaded a pregnancy app and read everything she could about signs of miscarriage and what to expect that first trimester.

"Frankly, I was obsessed," she said. "Every other thought was about this pregnancy and what was happening to my body."

When the cramping began, Kari went to her doctor to confirm her pregnancy wasn't ectopic, hoping to avoid the hospital. After speaking with her OB, she opted to let the fetus pass naturally. She knew more or less what to expect this time, including not to ask about psychosocial support since, once more, she was only eight weeks along.

She struggled again to get out of bed, but Jon was again able to coax her out of her funk. Still, she had a rough time returning to work. She was at a new job and its environment was the most dehumanizing she'd ever encountered. When she explained to her boss that she needed time off from the grind because of the loss, he was flippant. "Well, my mom had a bunch of miscarriages and then she had the four of us," he told her.

In other words, "Life goes on, now get back to work."

Kari exploded in laughter when she relayed her boss's callousness to me. It was all she could do not to pull her hair out at the memory. She knew he was implying that she should be hopeful; still, it was a drastic change from her last manager, who'd sent flowers and a card and asked if there was anything he could do.

This was the job where Kari found herself, shortly after the second miscarriage, helping the distressed woman deliver the baby girl left in the NICU. Seeing the newborn shake her perfect little fists, Kari felt a sense of helplessness and anger rising in her belly.

"I had so much love to give a child, there was a real yearning," she said, her voice growing louder. "How could God just let someone be a mother who didn't even want her child? It didn't seem fair."

Kari had waited a long time before having sex for the first time, and she had decided to hold off having kids until she got married. She'd always endeavored to do the right thing in God's eyes. Over the years she had stopped attending church, but she hadn't stopped believing.

"I used to read the Bible and pray every day, but I stopped after that miscarriage." Kari spoke with conviction. "I wouldn't say that I don't pray anymore, but the way I pray and what I consider prayer has changed."

Kari said she had lost touch with her spirituality, with a ritual of prayer that spoke to her authentic relationship with a higher power, well before the miscarriages. She had come to see a fallacy in praying for material things or for God to intervene on her behalf. Now her prayers were more humble, asking for guidance to be a better person.

"Maybe I needed this to happen to see things more in that perspective," Kari reflected. "Now when I'm faced with a challenge, it's like God helped me understand—God helped me to have love, not judgment, in this moment."

I asked what the experience was like for her and Jon as a couple.

"Oh God, it was difficult for him." Kari let out a long sigh. "I felt sorry for him because even though this was my second miscarriage, it was technically his third because of his first wife."

Jon was a man of few words, but when he used them they were thoughtful and purposeful, Kari explained.

"Baby," he told her, "at this point, you're my main concern. If it's just the two of us, I'm happy."

I felt my eyes well up at the tenderness Kari's voice conveyed as she shared those words. I wasn't entirely confident my own marriage could withstand a life without children.

"It was good to hear," Kari admitted. "You know, 'cause I did wonder if I was enough."

Kari felt her body had betrayed her. She recalled a haunting dream she'd had right before her first miscarriage, where she was trying to hold on to her baby but it kept slipping away. She cried out for help to get the baby's head up, then watched in horror as the slick body escaped her fumbling arms.

"I'm not that woo," Kari confided in her hairdresser at the time, "but is the spirit world trying to tell me something? Like maybe my body can't hold on to a baby?"

"Come on, now," the woman reassured her. "Everything will be fine, don't you worry."

After the second miscarriage, Kari wasn't so sure.

"It's a funny thing," she said with a shrug. "We started having sex again, but I wasn't really trying anymore to get pregnant. I'd adapted this mindset that we might not have children. My husband said I'm enough, so I stopped hoping."

Kari was having shoulder problems at the time and her doctor advised her to get surgery. She figured why not, considering she'd given up on trying to conceive. She scheduled the operation.

In the leadup to the procedure, she was shocked to receive a call from the orthopedist's office congratulating her on her pregnancy. The nurse explained that she'd have to postpone the surgery.

Kari hadn't missed a period yet, so it was early days.

"Jon was happy, as usual," Kari recalled, "and I was happy too, in a strange way, but also nervous."

Unlike her prior pregnancies, morning sickness wiped Kari off her feet this time. A good friend cheered her on, saying, "This is such a good sign! It might sound bad, but just keep feeling sick. I'm so happy for you!"

Kari, too, believed this one might be different. It felt different. But the anxiety was still omnipresent. At around eight weeks, Kari noticed some spotting and immediately called a medical hotline. A nurse explained that it was too early to do anything; she'd need to wait it out.

Kari took a day off work to lie in bed, expecting at any moment to start miscarrying. The next day, the spotting was gone but the nausea remained.

As the pregnancy progressed and they heard the heartbeat and saw the first sonograms, Kari became more hopeful. She trusted when the doctor said everything looked okay. After each healthy visit, Jon framed the ultrasound printout and proudly placed it on the mantle.

Those frames now boast photos of their six-year-old son, Carter.

Just six months after Carter was born, Kari learned she was pregnant again. Not only was she dealing with a newborn and a toxic work environment but Jon had also just lost his job, so finances were tight. When she miscarried within the week, she found herself uncomfortably relieved.

"As much as I wanted more children, the timing was terrible," she admitted. "I didn't fully mourn that loss, and to this day I feel guilty about my sense of relief."

Between pumping milk, dealing with the crazies at work, and putting food on the table, there wasn't much time to process the loss. Little Carter was a welcome distraction. Kari says she barely remembers the pain or her recovery from that third miscarriage.

The family moved cross-country to Oregon when Carter was a toddler, and Kari found herself adjusting to a new job and culture. She'd recently been diagnosed with Graves' disease, an autoimmune disorder that causes hyperthyroidism, so she had to contend with that on top of Carter, who now ran circles around her.

Kari suspected the thyroid issue might explain her many miscarriages, but her doctor's prognosis wasn't conclusive. Her prescribed medication contraindicated with pregnancy, but at this point, conception wasn't on her radar anyway.

Kari's condition went into remission after a few years, and soon enough she was pregnant again. During the first ultrasound, she noticed the heartbeat was low and went straight to worry. The nurses said they'd track it again when she came in the following week. Since she was now in her early forties, her doctors wanted to monitor the pregnancy closely.

That Kari had even seen a heartbeat gave her hope. In her earlier miscarriages, the fetus had never progressed that far. Plus, she had morning sickness, just like she'd had with Carter.

The couple made a big video announcement when Kari's parents were visiting from Maryland, and they giddily sent it to their immediate family. They decided to wait until after the first trimester to tell their son, however, because they knew the five-year-old would blab to anyone who'd listen. Carter wanted nothing more than a sibling.

"Every night when we'd say our prayers together, he'd always wish for a sister," Kari said. "So I really couldn't wait to tell him."

The day after they shared the video, Kari started spotting. Her mother prayed for her, insisting everything would be fine, while Kari made an appointment with her OB. When she went in, the heartbeat was silent and Kari's spirits were crushed.

She passed the fetal tissue naturally over the next two days. Fortunately, her mother could help with Carter and the housework. There was so much going on for Kari professionally that she snapped right back to work and teaching classes. In hindsight, she said, that was a mistake.

"I wasn't bringing my best self. When I looked back on my evaluations, they were brutal." Kari's voice was sluggish. I could sense her shame. "People said I was hostile, and I'd never seen that in an evaluation before. I really should have taken time off to care for myself."

Kari's boss was refreshingly empathetic. She helped arrange for her to take a leave and encouraged her to seek counseling through the human resources department. Through her OB practice, Kari got connected with a social worker—and was blown away by the power of therapy.

"It was incredibly cathartic to talk with a counselor." Kari's voice cracked. "Just cried my eyes out." She paused to wipe her nose. "I kept going back to my first miscarriage and how that was still impacting me."

Kari couldn't shake the abandonment and despair of her hospital visit years earlier. Nor could she forget the reaction she'd gotten from her Black OB when she asked for the very support she was finally receiving.

She told her counselor in the suburban Northwest practice, "I'm so grateful this practice offered me help without me having to ask."

I asked if there was anything missing from her care there.

"I would have loved to have been surrounded by other women of color who'd gone through it," Kari said, then drew in a sharp breath. "I know that's difficult living here," in her largely white suburb, "but I definitely would've appreciated that."

Being so far from family and friends, she missed the hugs and easy conversation she was used to with her Black sisters.

"There's something about the support that Black women give one another," Kari explained. "Not to say I don't have wonderful, supportive white friends, but having the support of another Black woman is so different, so therapeutic."

During an aftercare visit, some nurses told Kari that the most fertile time to conceive was in the months following a miscarriage. After discussing the issue at length, she and Jon decided to go for it. Kari was forty-three, Jon nearly fifty. They were exhausted with all the loss, but seduced by the vision of growing their family. It was their last hurrah.

The nurses' wisdom prevailed: Kari quickly got pregnant. Only this time, there was no morning sickness, and the initial ultrasound showed a slightly small sac. Kari had a bad feeling.

"I didn't allow myself to have hope, because I'd had it with the last miscarriage when it had a heartbeat, and I wanted to protect myself from that pain."

Sure enough, at the cursed eight weeks, Kari lost the pregnancy. She and Jon were despondent.

This time, Kari took longer off work, but she mostly spent it caring for her son. Jon was back at a new job, and the days seemed to fill up without any time for reflection.

When Kari returned to work, she could barely pull it together. She didn't understand why she was having such a hard time. The depression weighed on her for weeks before she sought support again.

Kari's therapist pushed her to work through her grief—not to merely scratch the surface but to complete the process of grieving. Kari hadn't connected her depression to the miscarriages until she began talking through her feelings.

As part of her therapy, Kari kept a journal and wrote letters to her unborn children. It comforted her to imagine them all waiting somewhere for her—not in Heaven, per se (she was careful to let me know that), but some spiritual realm she alone had conceived. Her therapist also encouraged her to talk with a friend who'd had a miscarriage within weeks of Kari's, which proved symbiotic for both women's grieving and healing.

Kari was not having another baby, but she and Jon still wanted to grow the family, so they opted for a Chiweenie. Kari discovered a new form of healing through puppy care. Her son, meanwhile, was over the moon.

One night shortly after Prince and his purple leashes arrived in their home, while Kari and her son were saying their prayers, Carter leaned toward his mom and whispered, "Prince is kinda like my baby brother, so I'm not gonna pray for a baby sister anymore."

Knowing she wasn't letting her little man down, Kari felt a huge weight lift from her chest.

I wanted to hear more about Carter and Prince and being Black in white Oregon, but our time was running out. When I asked what advice Kari had for other women experiencing loss, she was quick to answer.

"Don't ever let other people diminish your experience," she asserted. "People act as if you don't make it a big deal, then it's not a big deal. But they don't realize the harm, because if it happens again, it's just stacks upon stacks upon stacks until you're so deep in the grief you can barely function."

Kari urged women to ignore the message to sweep things under the rug and put on a happy face. Get support and honor your grief, she said.

"Don't torture yourself like I did."

CHAPTER 6

Abby

"Nobody walks you through the finances of loss."

THE SIX-YEAR-OLD FASTENED her blond braids with pastel ribbons she'd found on the sidewalk and set out rummaging around the house for anything festive. She found some craft supplies and old party favors tucked away in her older sister's half of the bedroom closet—silly things her sister would never use but had hidden from her out of spite, a punishment for Abby's goody two-shoes tendency to spend hours repurposing odds and ends only to go and give it all away.

It was Good Friday and Abby knew most households on her street wouldn't be getting Easter baskets. It was the same story every year. Her family lived on food stamps and her mother, with her dad long out of the picture, struggled to make ends meet. The whole neighborhood was scraping by, but Abby was determined to make the holiday special. On Sunday morning, she'd take whatever she'd collected, add some fresh grass and a hand-painted plastic egg she'd saved from last year, and put it on the doorstep of every kid on the block.

Abby knew from the get-go she wanted to have at least six kids. She'd given up on bonding with her sister and always longed for more siblings. Her maternal instincts kicked in well before puberty.

"I started caring for children very young. I would just gather the kids and we'd play school, house, store—whatever I created for them," Abby, now forty-three, recalled as she sat across from me cross-legged on my sofa, dressed sporty-casual in muted hues, the morning sunlight entering through my sliding deck doors dancing on her rounded shoulders. She looked like the sort of kindly neighbor I could bother for a cup of sugar without feeling intrusive. While not effusive, she had a friendly, reliable presence, and an uncanny resemblance to the singer-songwriter Liz Phair.

As much as Abby enjoyed mothering her younger neighbors and excelled at school, her upbringing had left some scars.

"Financially, it scared the living daylights out of me," Abby told me. "I knew I never wanted to have a family go through what I went through."

Her husband Mark, whom she met when she was twenty-one, also had a rough childhood: he was an only child, and his mother was emotionally abusive. For him, the thought of starting a family was daunting. He was on board to eventually have a big family with Abby, but it was going to take some time for his confidence to match his heart.

As Abby got older and friends became parents, she satisfied her mothering yen by tending to their children. By the time she and Mark felt financially and emotionally secure enough to think seriously about conceiving, she was thirty-seven.

Some years earlier, Abby had decided to go off the pill in an effort to make her life more natural, so there was no period of adjustment when they stopped using birth control—they got pregnant right away. Abby focused her exhilaration at the news into sensing into her changing body's needs and researching an OB for their first prenatal visit.

"We saw an early heartbeat, at six weeks," Abby said excitedly, "which they tell you is a good indication, right? That if you see a heartbeat, the likelihood of miscarriage is very small."

The next week, Abby started having cramps and light spotting. Not one to panic, she pragmatically called her doctor and was told to come right in.

I noticed Abby's hands searching for something to do before they settled on tightening her blond ponytail. She flashed a quick smile at her two-year-old daughter, Dakota, who'd just erupted in hungry giggles opening a bag of cheddar bunnies on the coffee table, before turning back to me and letting out a long sigh.

She recapped the visit in strictly clinical terms: "The heartbeat was gone."

An inventory management professional in the SF Bay Area, Abby is a self-described feminist. She didn't harbor any of the shame so many women suffer in the aftermath of pregnancy loss. She already knew people who had miscarried and her doctor was careful to reiterate how common it was, that she shouldn't feel alone.

"That was reassuring," Abby shared, "but then when you get back home, you start to Google."

After doing some research online, Abby jotted down a list of tests she thought she might need. When she called her OB on a late Friday afternoon, the doctor was cautiously supportive.

"I'd be happy to run any tests," she told Abby, "but honestly I think it was a fluke. There's no reason not to expect a positive outcome next time."

Abby still wasn't sure how she wanted to cleanse her body of the pregnancy. Her OB had warned her that letting it pass naturally could take up to six weeks, but she wanted to research more on her own before deciding whether to go with the D&C.

"Call me over the weekend if you change your mind," the OB said. She gave Abby her cell phone number and encouraged her to use it if she wanted to go with the misoprostol pill instead.

Abby had heard that acupuncture could help with miscarriage by stimulating the onset of labor. After reading more online, she called the perinatal acupuncturist who'd performed labor induction treatment on her sister and cousins. When Abby told her what was happening, the practitioner told her to come right over. She stayed open late on a Saturday to treat her.

"By evening, I felt everything cramping and tense, just extremely painful," Abby recalled. "I happen to have a crazy high pain tolerance. It must be hereditary, my mom and sister do too. And it was still super painful!" She laughed. "Thankfully, it was over quickly." She passed everything that night.

Abby and Mark were eager to get pregnant again. Her OB told them they could start right away, but her acupuncturist had a different take: Chinese medicine says to wait three full cycles before trying again. For Abby, the choice was clear.

"It was helpful to have my acupuncturist, who deals with pregnancy loss all day, every day," Abby explained. "Whereas the OBs— it's not necessarily something they see on a daily basis."

While they waited, Abby regularly received acupuncture to help heal her mind and body—"all the good stuff that acupuncture does," she said, glowing. She paused and Dakota grew quiet, looking up from her busy fingers to her mother. "In hindsight, I don't know if I would have accepted that same advice. I wish I'd tried sooner, 'cause there was more loss to come and I already felt the clock ticking."

Abby was pregnant four months after the miscarriage. This time, she did more research about where she wanted to give birth and narrowed in on a medical center that shared her natural-minded values of midwife participation. This meant leaving the OB she loved, but she figured it was worth it.

She made her first appointment for ten weeks, knowing she couldn't bear the disappointment of not hearing a heartbeat on the second visit. As she grew bigger, she was heartened to experience classic pregnancy symptoms, but soon they tapered off. As they did, her usual cool was replaced by anxiety.

"I couldn't make sense of all the doubt. Like, *is* there anything real behind this?" Abby was at the edge of the couch, shaking her head. "Mind tricks you start to play on yourself."

When they went in, they found no heartbeat and a fetus measuring what would be expected at eight weeks, not ten. Yet Abby showed no signs of miscarriage. Since the staff was concerned her body wouldn't take care of passing the fetus naturally, they recommended she have a D&C. They even offered to take her into the room next door to have one right then and there.

"I was shocked by that," Abby recalled, sitting back.

She refused. She wanted to see her acupuncturist before she considered anything else.

She received acupuncture later that day, but the treatment didn't trigger anything. She waited three days, got acupuncture again—still nothing.

"If nothing happens in a week," the acupuncturist advised, "I want you to go back to your OB. Not clearing it means risking an infection, which would be awful."

Days later, Abby began to feel the familiar pains of cramping. At first, she was relieved to know the needles were finally working; before long, however, the pain had gotten so bad she was vomiting. She didn't think she could take any more. Begrudgingly, she called the OB's office to let them know she was ready for the D&C.

"Sorry, we're all booked today," the nurse told her, "and tomorrow's Thanksgiving, so . . ."

"Well, I . . ." Abby was dumbfounded. "What exactly do you do with someone in my situation?"

"Oh, we'll just schedule you after the weekend, and if it gets so bad you can't wait 'til Monday, get yourself to the ER."

"Wait . . . What?!" Abby squeaked, relaying her reaction to this conversation.

Dakota doubled over in laughter, thinking her mom had cracked a joke.

Abby smiled her way—"Yes, sweetie, your mom sounds a bit crazy, right?"—but when she turned toward me again, her fire instantly reignited. "I was just so taken aback that they would tell someone that." Her face reddened. "It really turned me off to that practice."

Mark's family was expecting them for the holiday meal. Abby's sheer grit carried her through Thanksgiving and into the weekend without having to visit a hospital.

By Monday, when they were driving to the clinic for the procedure, Abby was cramping and bleeding so heavily, she thought she might already be clearing it.

She told them this when she arrived, and they sent her to the restroom with a plastic cup to collect the tissue; with a sample, they could test the likelihood of Abby having similar issues in the future. When Abby handed them the sample, however, they said there was no tissue—that she must not have passed it yet. So they wheeled her into a room for the D&C.

After a brief pre-op exam, the doctor set down her speculum and slid back on her stool.

"Actually, your body's in the process of getting rid of it right now," she said, explaining that Abby's cervix was wide open. "Either I can go in there and finish the job, or you can."

Abby sighed. Her preference to go it naturally was well established; she was worried about scar tissue with the surgery.

"Honestly, it's all right here," her doctor reassured her. "You'll probably pass it by this evening."

Back at home, Abby spent the night clutching her belly and waiting for the pain to end. When she rose from her half-slumber the following morning with an intense urge to pee, she barely made it to the toilet before a rush of a mass passed through her, releasing her from her agony.

"That was the hardest miscarriage, physically and mentally." Abby shuddered with the memory. "The back and forth—you've passed it, no you haven't passed it. The physical pain and then the doom of testing they sent me through."

Given Abby's age, her doctor decided to run the gamut of genetic tests. With her low blood pressure, the poking, prodding, and countless vials seemed to take hours.

The results came back normal.

After another three months of acupuncture, Abby was pregnant again.

Feeling the last OB practice had failed her, Abby asked around for recommendations for a different doctor. A nurse friend of hers who'd been trying to conceive for a number of years referred Abby to her Swedish OB who ran a practice with his partner. "They're almost like midwives; trust me, you'll be in great hands," she assured her.

Abby made an appointment with the OB's partner for six weeks gestation—office policy.

In everyone's excitement to see the heartbeat, the new OB wanted Abby to get another slew of tests and make sure Mark was tested as well to rule him out as negatively impacting the genetic makeup. She prescribed her an anti-inflammatory diet, along with a regimen of probiotic progesterone. Though Abby wasn't thrilled about all the blood work, she trusted her new doctor and her naturopathic approach.

Abby never experienced morning sickness and was slow to gain weight in the second trimester. With each dreaded appointment, she wondered if things would be okay. Every bodily change was an alarm bell.

"I *loved* being pregnant," she said dreamily. "But it's hard to enjoy pregnancy when you've been through what I've been through."

Mark was coping with his own doubts and fears about losing another pregnancy.

"He was nerve-racked," Abby recalled. "But he's calm by nature, and so am I, so it was okay. We didn't feed off each other."

They hesitated to tell people about the pregnancy too early; they'd learned the hard way with the first two miscarriages. When they made it to twenty weeks, they decided to announce. But it was only when they reached the benchmark that meant the pregnancy would be viable outside the womb—twenty-eight weeks—that Abby was finally able to relax.

Baby Charles arrived just two weeks shy of his due date through a smoothly facilitated, natural birth. Abby pushed for almost three hours, determined to deliver on her own.

"I didn't want *anyone* telling me I was having a C-section!" she howled.

Abby had by now faced the music that six kids were out of the question; she and Mark were set on staying in the Bay Area, and there was no way they could afford such a big family there. "I wasn't about to move to a farm to have sex," she said, laughing.

I chuckled, impressed she could weave humor into such wrenching stories of loss. I wondered if her emotional cool was for the daughter doing mini-somersaults beside her, or if this was just Abby being Abby.

When I asked if she ever sought counseling after the losses, she described her friends as largely inexperienced with miscarriage but sympathetic listeners.

"I wouldn't say I'm closed off emotionally but . . . we just never talked about feelings growing up."

Abby saw this as a generational issue, but I sensed it had more to do with her upbringing. When I floated that idea, she agreed.

"Sure, I had to grow up so early; I felt it was my job to get myself well and not be a wreck about this kind of thing."

As kind and emotionally intelligent as I found her, Abby was far from warm and fuzzy. I imagined the stoic little girl watching neighbors' kids in the way she brushed off my comments speaking to the difficulty of her losses. But this is exactly what women and mothers so often do. We're quick to care for others but always the first to pick ourselves up, brush off the dirt, and keep forging ahead.

For Abby, this wasn't a concern about being burdensome or needy. It was the independence she'd learned at a young age that was so crucial to her resilience and well-being; it was just who she was.

Now nearly thirty-nine, Abby knew that even if six kids was out of the question, she wanted at least one more baby. She got her period back when Charles was eleven months old and was pregnant by her next cycle. Because of her advanced age and history, she went in between five and six weeks for her first prenatal visit. The ultrasound showed a fertilized egg but no heartbeat. The OB said not to worry, as every pregnancy was different.

When they returned in the advised ten days, the news was the same. The pregnancy was over.

My God, Abby thought, *are we gonna go through this all over again?!*

Her rebound from this miscarriage was much quicker, primarily because this time there was a child clamoring for her attention—an experience shared by many grieving parents. She was grateful that Charles was still nursing; she found the activity comforted her (arguably more than it did her newborn!). Spending time with him inspired her confidence as a mother, someone with the wondrous power to create another life.

"I knew it was possible because here's the living proof." Abby glanced at Dakota, playfully untangling herself from under a blanket, then dropped to a half-whisper. "But now I've got my fucking forties looming!" She threw her hands in the air.

Three months later, Abby was pregnant again. The technology had improved significantly, so they were able to run genetic tests even earlier—"Science is amazing!" Abby cheered—but the genetic screening came back inconclusive. Abby again took to Google, where the overriding opinion was "bad news." She was able to wrangle the test results directly from the genetics company, but she'd have to wait a few days to make sense of them at her fourteen-week visit.

At the visit the ultrasound technician was all business—an attitude that stoked both Abby and Mark's fears. She took measurements and photos, then left to get the doctor.

"Bedside manners are not her cup of tea. It's kind of known about her." Abby would never forget the technician. "But my OB, whom I just adore, really values her due diligence and expertise."

The doctor burst through the door. "Well, this isn't good," she greeted them.

Abby immediately started crying.

"Let me show you what I'm seeing." Her OB put the ultrasound back up. "Here's all the fluid. You're measuring four times what we would consider okay." She looked carefully at Abby. "There's no doubt in my mind that this is trisomy, and it's one of the worst cases I've seen."

Trisomy means there's a third chromosome in the body's cells instead of the normal two.

As the OB listed each visible deformity on the ultrasound, Abby wondered if what she heard was actually happening. Could her doctor be wrong? The inconclusive results suddenly made sense.

"I would recommend you terminate right away," the OB said, then gave them the stats: 5 percent of trisomy babies make it to term, and of those only 1 percent live beyond one year[8].

Abby couldn't fathom going through with the pregnancy.

"With our current situation, already having a family, and then financially and emotionally—I just couldn't," she explained to me. "And my age! If we wanted another baby, I'd be, ugh, too many years old!"

Abby's doctor ushered her and Mark into another room with a genetics specialist, who began scribbling numbers on a piece of paper, calculating their genetic odds with those Punnett squares she'd learned back in high school biology.

"Here are your chances," she told them. "This is your age, this is . . ."

It was all a blur, but by the end of it, Abby and Mark had made a decision.

The soonest the staff could get Abby in to terminate was in two days.

"Here I was, going to have a D&C, which I never thought in a million years would happen to me!" Abby recalled.

She and Mark cried from the ultrasound appointment to their front door. When they called to break the news to close friends and family, they could barely manage words. Emboldened by the successful pregnancy with Charles, they'd announced this pregnancy at eleven weeks—a decision they now deeply regretted.

On top of the grief, Abby worried how Mark's mother would react to their electing not to carry the baby to term. She feared the family's conservative views on abortion would prevent her mother-in-law from feeling empathy toward them. She didn't want to feel judged or to seed any friction in the family.

Luckily, her fears didn't come to pass. "Once his mom read up on it, she was like, 'Holy moly, this is not good!'" Abby said. "We're not talking Down Syndrome. We're talking massive deformities."

Abby and Mark cried all the way to the procedure.

"I remember Mark holding my hand, and then they made him leave for the anesthesia, and tears just running down my face."

The nurse even cried with Abby. Everyone's emotions were high.

She had wanted to be awake for the procedure, but her OB refused. "You're better going under," she told her.

"The martyr part of me wanted to be awake for it. I wanted to see it." Abby's frame softened. "I'm glad I didn't do it, though. I don't know how I'd be after . . ."

Abby took ten days to recover in the comfort of her home. She had no interest in showing up to her job waddling around in giant pads. "Who wants to deal with all that?" she complained. "No one talks about that stuff—how awkward and uncomfortable it is, and what you need in recovery."

Her boss encouraged her to take the time; true to Abby's nature, however, she ended up working many of those days.

Abby and Mark were still hopeful for another child. With the trauma of the last loss weighing heavily on their hearts, they were terrified to try again. Abby was nearing forty and the chances of having another trisomy had only grown with time. Her doctor was clear about the increased risk but encouraged them to give it another go.

Three months later, they were pregnant again. Once the genetic tests came back normal, Abby breathed a quick sigh of relief. But she wasn't feeling the baby moving around in her belly. She couldn't shake the fear that something could go wrong at any moment.

As the anxiety continued into the third trimester, a dear friend who'd lost her six-year-old son told Abby about an energy worker who'd helped her find peace and solace. She insisted that Abby see her.

The healer reassured her the pregnancy would go well, and told her that she sensed strong female energy from the womb. The thought of having a baby girl lifted Abby's spirits.

The doctors threatened induction when Abby was almost at forty weeks, but she put her foot down.

"There was no way I'd let them induce me," Abby proclaimed. By then, she felt in tune with her body and knew what it was telling her.

True to the energy worker's premonition, Abby gave birth right on her due date—to the lovely little blonde spilling cheddar bunnies on my Turkish rug. I paused for a moment to take in the joyful toddler, so unaware of the preciousness of her existence.

When I asked Abby about the role of alternative medicine and healing in her motherhood journey, she immediately spoke to how fortunate she was to be able to afford quality care.

It was clear how physically and emotionally taxing losing a pregnancy could be, she said, but what about the financial piece? The double taboo of death and money is rarely discussed, from healthcare providers and insurance companies to family and friends. Most pregnant women don't stop to consider, let alone budget for, the out-of-pocket expenses they might incur in case of a loss. Most of us would just as soon forget those painful, often unexpected, fees.

While most insurance companies won't cover expenses for alternative treatments, Abby was fortunate to have decent health insurance through her employer—but, "It still was super expensive. I just thought, through that entire process, why am I having to pay to go through this pain? It's so unfair!"

She felt that women having to pay out of pocket for painful and traumatic experiences was just another symptom of a broken healthcare system. She suggested that pregnancy loss expenses should be a pass for women.

"*Clearly*, a man wrote the insurance coverage for these procedures!" she said, fuming. "Nobody walks you through the finances of loss. But why not?"

The financial burden is exacerbated for women who don't get paid time off (PTO), or don't feel they can broach the sensitive subject with their bosses.

"No one tells you that when you work full time, you have to share your miscarriage experience in order to get your PTO. Otherwise, they'll think something weird is going on."

Women should get proper medical leave and at least a bit of sympathy, she said. "Not a 'You've been gone a week, here's all this work to do' kind of thing."

Abby considered herself incredibly fortunate. Her direct boss's sister had just gone through something similar, which allowed them to develop a shared bond. Her job also allowed her the flexibility to work from home.

"Think about all these women who work in law offices or banking who can't leave," she said. "They're chained to their desks because the work never stops. My gosh, how do these people even deal?"

One of her coworkers was training to be a volunteer doula at SF General and enlightened Abby to the existence of doulas who support women through miscarriage—a wonderful resource, albeit one limited to a relatively small number of practices. Abby didn't feel she needed that for herself in any of her four miscarriages, but now she regularly suggests it to others.

Circling back to my question about alternative medicine, Abby stressed the importance of self-advocacy and research. "You need people in your court that are willing to go to bat for you, and the OB community isn't there," she lamented. "It's shocking there's none of that support at the OB office, no mental check-in. Especially if you've never had a baby or miscarriage before." Acknowledging the financial difficulties many would-be mothers and families are up against, she nevertheless stressed the importance of lining up a doula, an acupuncturist, a chiropractor, a caring OB—a whole team of people to offer support. Most importantly, she said, women must surround themselves with other women who've been through something similar to help protect against feelings of isolation.

In her case, she said, the losses she suffered revealed her own strength to her.

"I already knew I was pretty capable, coming from what I came from, but much more so now." Abby smiled, taking a reflective pause, before concluding, "The female body's pretty darn remarkable."

I considered Abby's fierce strength and martyrdom as she nearly forced herself to stay awake for her trisomy D&C. Why do we strain and sacrifice ourselves to such extremes? As women and mothers, do we not already endure enough with every menstrual cycle, every pregnancy, every child, every loss? We don't have to be martyrs to be strong.

CHAPTER 7

Rae

"We remade our lives around this."

"RAFAELA, LOVE, let your brother gather his own mangos."

The wiry, pigtailed girl promptly jumped from the trunk of the towering tree, scrunched up her nose, and stomped her foot with feigned disappointment.

"Thank you, dear." Rae lifted her sunglasses to wink at her frisky daughter.

The Morong morning was bright and balmy. She listened to the waves gently lap onto shore, a soft breeze ruffling the palm fronds above her.

The screen door creaked open as Colin brought out mackerel, eggs, and spicy jicama salad. Rafaela clapped her hands and Caio cheered with gleeful anticipation of Saturday brunch. Rae left her book on the lounge chair and glided toward the lanai, where Colin greeted her with a cold green coconut, straw drilled into its top, and a kiss on the cheek.

This was Rae's happy place, as she so beautifully painted it for me over our Skype call, a wistful look in her damp eyes. While the Philippines proved a stepstone along their journey, that happy place was an elusive fantasy Rae and Colin chased for years, well after their time near Manila came to a close.

Rae's Filipino family had welcomed them with open arms. Come, they'd said after the wedding. Come, do your freelance work with your American dollar–paying clients and live with us here on the beach. We'll spoil our future grandkids while you work. You'll see, they'll have an enchanted island life. Just come.

Rae and Colin, then thirty-year-old newlyweds and business partners, didn't have many reasons to stay in Oakland. Their consulting business was winding down, they were mostly working from home, and it felt absurd to pay such an astronomical rent for their cramped apartment.

"We don't really need to be here," Rae said, describing their thinking at the time. "All of our clients are on Skype. Like, wow, wouldn't it be hard to have kids here, anyway? They could come at any moment!" Playing to their romantic naïveté, Rae theatrically batted her brown eyes at Colin, who sat supportively by his wife during our chat. "We could get spontaneously pregnant any day now!" The couple half laughed, half sighed.

They were confident they'd get pregnant when they started casually trying in May 2014.

Rae visited her Ob/Gyn, excited to discuss her and Colin's procreative plans—only to get abnormal results on her pap smear.

Soon after, Rae had to undergo LEEP surgery, where a thin wire loop carrying a high-frequency current removes abnormal cells in the cervix (it's not unlike freezing off a skin tag). Her body needed six months to heal before she and Colin could try to conceive again.

In late summer 2015, after eight months of leisurely trying to get pregnant, Rae and Colin packed up for the Philippines in the hopes of soon having a baby.

The couple tracked Rae's ovulation for the first six months abroad. When they still didn't conceive, they grew quietly anxious about why. Rae met with an OB, who confirmed her fallopian tubes were open, then started on the fertility drug Clomid, followed by several ovulation stimulants. Her doctor suggested intrauterine insemination (IUI) down the road if the oral meds didn't work.

Every month Rae's period arrived, her fear and disappointment took on greater proportions. "I had to talk myself down," she confessed. "Like, I'm still young, it'll be fine."

Except it didn't feel fine. She was anxious to move on to the next, more powerful tool in the fertility tool box.

When they advanced to IUI, a nurse checked the follicle growth and advised them when to have sex. Rae and Colin were hypervigilant each round they tried. Still, they couldn't catch a break.

They gave themselves some time off from Project Baby and booked an overseas trip for the summer. "Everyone said we'd go to Europe and get spontaneously pregnant," Rae recalled, shaking her head.

I nodded passionately as Rae grumbled about family members who had insisted she and Colin were trying too hard.

"Just relax," I commiserated, recalling my own frustration hearing loved ones brush aside my fertility concerns. "Nature has its way."

"Yes!" Rae balled her fists in the air. "That frustrated me to no end, but a part of me believed it might be true." A part of her needed it to be true. "I thought, *Great, we'll drink wine, it'll be romantic. We'll be in the City of Love—of course we'll get pregnant!*" She leaned forward and exhaled the words, "Well, that totally didn't happen."

When they returned to the Philippines from their idyllic European vacation in the fall of 2016, they determined it was time to take the plunge with in-vitro fertilization (IVF).

Rae felt IVF was a huge leap, but the natural next step. They'd already exhausted the available options and, more importantly, in the Philippines the procedure was just a fraction of the cost of what they would've had to shell out in the US.

"There's been so much about IVF in the media—movies on Netflix, a six-part podcast, influencers and regular people on Instagram and Facebook—I feel like it's everywhere," Rae said. "But it's happening on a much bigger scale in the States." She and Colin didn't know anyone in the Philippines who had done it. But there, IVF wasn't cost-prohibitive. They didn't have to mortgage a house or dip into retirement. So they didn't agonize over it like so many couples do in the US, forced to plan around limited finances and rigid work schedules. Their work and living situations were entirely flexible.

Rae's aunt connected the couple with a doctor friend from medical school. Since they knew there wasn't much IVF done in the Philippines, they didn't bother researching other clinicians. They were impatient to move forward.

Rae did everything conceivable to make the transfer procedure as seamless as possible. She had a great night's sleep the night before, ate a hearty breakfast the morning of, and got acupuncture just before heading to the clinic.

Despite her best efforts, a frenetic, anxious energy seemed to have taken hold of her doctor and his assistant, bursting Rae's bubble of calm.

"A little to the left!" the OB hissed.

"No, to the right!" snapped the sonographer, a bead of sweat forming on her brow.

"No, no. We need to go left!" The OB's voice was rising. "The other left!"

Rae was conscious throughout the exchange. The clinicians only had ten minutes to complete the transfer with any chance of success. The clock was ticking. Loudly.

"There I am, trying to visualize my happy baby, and my medical team is at each other's throats," Rae shared, rolling her eyes. "It didn't instill a lot of confidence."

Rae's doctor likely wasn't comfortable performing IVF because it wasn't in high demand, either in the clinic or the country.

"It was a traumatic first transfer experience." Rae made a sad face and shrugged.

She was initially hopeful when she tested positive afterward, but her HCG rose only slightly, then fell.

"I guess that would be the first miscarriage," Colin observed. He and Rae were seated at a desk, a thick notebook spread open before them. They were flipping through it during our call, trying to match up specific details to a timeline. "Yep, miscarriage number one."

After the failed transfer, the OB recommended Rae have a hysteroscopy to check for polyps or other abnormalities. The same tech's lack of ease and experience again presented challenges.

"She couldn't navigate my cervix, and I'm like, you just did a transfer, but you can't . . . !" Rae's jaw dropped.

The technician openly complained that Rae's cervix was too tight, suggesting that the LEEP scarring was preventing her from getting any decent images. (In reality, the scarring, which was minimal, shouldn't have impacted the hysteroscopy.)

"So you were essentially blamed for the technician's incompetence?" I asked, noting an uncomfortable appreciation for my own relatively respectful, if uneventful, experience of fertility care.

Rae responded with a simple "pfft."

Meanwhile, Colin was in the waiting room, expecting Rae to come out shortly. That sort of imaging was normally a routine fifteen-minute procedure. He waited six hours.

"Worst experience ever," Rae muttered.

"All of our experiences in that hospital were traumatic," Colin said.

"And it's the nicest hospital!" Rae piped in.

Renowned in the Philippines for its quality of care, the hospital resembled an upscale hotel, with valet parking and a pianist in the lobby, and it attracted patients from far and wide, including foreign diplomats.

Rae never booked the pricier private rooms, so she was shown to a locker room to get changed when she went in for procedures.

"It did *not* feel clean," she remarked with disgust. And, she said, because she wasn't on a gynecology wing, not just women but also men roamed the halls in loose gowns—not the intimate setting she'd hoped for, especially for the IVF transfer.

She cried for a full day when she returned home after the hysteroscopy, deflated by the disastrous, impersonal care as much as the failed transfer.

"The whole infertility thing was sinking in." Rae's frame sank, too, with the memory. "I really thought we were going to get it on our first try. We'd done everything else."

Within a week of the failed transfer, Rae called her stepdad in Brazil. As a physician, he understood the poor healthcare Rae was up against in the Philippines. He urged her to fly to São Paulo with Colin to do another hysteroscopy. While she was there, they'd do a round of IVF and a thorough physical to see if there were other health issues at play.

Since work remained flexible and IVF costs were comparable to the Philippines, if not cheaper, in Brazil, they decided to go for it.

"Most of the 10 to 15 percent of women who struggle with infertility also struggle with the finances," Rae—who threw herself into researching their new path to parenthood during that time—informed me. "Health insurance generally doesn't cover fertility care, let alone IVF."

While most couples don't have the flexibility or the finances to consider it, many are willing to uproot their lives so they can afford the gold-standard, and often last-hope, treatment. Traveling became a defining part of Rae and Colin's Project Baby experience.

"We remade our lives around infertility," Rae said—though she also said that if she didn't happen to have family in the Philippines and Brazil, she and Colin probably wouldn't have considered either for IVF. And after her experience in Manila, she advised friends to avoid it for any health-related matters.

"I realized I'd done that first IVF without checking everything," Rae explained. She felt that was common, especially in the States, where they don't look at the patient holistically. "If the cost wasn't so prohibitive or women's health so stigmatized and fucked up . . ." She sighed.

"That's a whole other book!" I cracked, producing a titter from Colin.

Rae bemoaned the lack of awareness and information about accessibility of IVF outside the US. In Brazil, a cycle cost them $4,000; with meds, $5,000. Had they stayed in the Bay Area, that would've been upwards of $20,000. On average, women in the US spend $12,000 per cycle, plus $1,500 to $3,000 on meds. No matter how you slice it, the differential is substantial—and that's just for one round. Many couples are not successful on the first or second or even third attempt.[9]

"IVF is more a sales product than actual care," Rae professed.

"A far cry from the holistic healthcare you were seeking," I suggested.

She bobbed her head in agreement.

In the US, Rae argued, where patients pay a premium for IVF, profits prevail over holistic medicine, without the guarantee of getting to enjoy the expensive end product: a baby. She recounted an analogy she heard in a documentary that resonated strongly with both her and Colin: "You have your sights set on a new car and tell the seller you'll give him $20,000 for it. The seller says, 'Okay, I'll flip a coin, and if it's heads I'll give you the car; tails, I'll just take your money. Either way, I'm keeping your twenty grand.'" She balked. "Nobody would do that! But that's basically IVF."

Motivated by the promise of better medical attention in Brazil, Rae began mapping out their trip. She would immediately get on the pill and stop taking it just before their flight so that her period would sync up perfectly with the cycle of ovarian stimulation. Next would be the egg "pickup," or retrieval, through outpatient surgery, at which time Colin would provide a fresh sperm sample for fertilization in the lab. While the viable embryo was forming, Rae would get a proper hysteroscopy and checkup. She'd have her next period, then do the embryo transfer, stat. It was a tight schedule.

"It actually went pretty well," Rae said. "Compared to the first one, it was a peaceful, successful transfer." She glanced at Colin, snickering. "'Successful' as in, you get it in there!"

After the transfer, the couple decided to wait things out somewhere they knew the language and had a comfortable place to stay. It was a direct flight from São Paulo to New York, so they hopped on a redeye and squatted at Rae's mother's flat in Manhattan. Her mother lived in Ohio and occasionally spent weekends in the City, so the place was pretty much theirs whenever they wanted.

"Honestly, it was nice to escape that heat. Plus, in New York, there's Chinese, Vietnamese, Thai, Filipino . . . which, there's none of in Brazil."

Rae was serious about her comfort foods.

A few weeks into their New York trip in June 2017, Rae got a positive pregnancy test, but within the week her HCG fell. She'd been pregnant nearly five weeks.

"Miscarriage number two," Colin remarked.

Rae corrected him; it was her third. She'd miscarried in her twenties, before they were together, and she'd also had an abortion in her teens. Neither had dramatically upset her life; she hadn't been remotely interested in having a baby then. But she was hellbent on it now.

I wondered how Rae coped with the losses. The impression I was getting was one of resilience and fortitude, with a whiff of nonchalance.

"The ones we told you about so far I would call small," Rae answered. "Wow, that sounds totally insensitive," she added, covering her mouth.

"When you say small, does that also refer to how you were feeling?" I asked.

"Yeah, emotionally small." Rae looked inquisitively at Colin.

"But the emotional buildup was always big," he said with a gentle smile.

Rae's an extremely open person, but when she tried talking with her friends about the loss, she found herself shutting down the moment they said something that wasn't 100 percent supportive. She started a fake Instagram account (Finsta) so she could share her experiences anonymously. Connecting with other women battling infertility and IVF was a huge source of support after the first losses, but the Finsta lost its healing power in the face of more difficult challenges to come.

Back in Brazil, Rae's doctors sprang into problem-solving mode. The hysteroscopy looked fine, so they ordered a host of autoimmune tests to look for any natural killer cells. They were concerned Rae might have an immune disorder that was attacking the fetus and impeding implantation, which would've been consistent with the pattern she was showing—a spike in HCG that then rapidly fell—but the tests came back normal. So in July 2017, it was onto Round Three.

For nearly two years, the couple cycled through dealing with Rae's health for forty-five to sixty days in Brazil, waiting out the pregnancy results in New York, and then—if it was a positive result—flying back to Brazil for the eight-week ultrasound.

"The treatments here were intense, so it was nice to get out of the country and take a break." Rae had begun to associate the whole of Brazil with IVF. "Everyone would ask, 'Have you traveled? Been to the beach?'" She laughed. "We didn't go to the beach for a year and a half!"

During the third round, the doctors discovered Rae was hyper-stimulating, meaning the fertility meds had overdone it hormonally on the ovaries. They experimented with lower and lower dosages to find the right balance—then had to cancel the round because they'd reduced the meds so much that Rae's ovaries couldn't make enough follicles to warrant the pickup.

"I totally remember this math, because if there were one or two follicles, they would let us have sex and try on our own." Rae's pedagogic tone projected confidence. "But if there were three or four follicles, then it was too many to safely have sex because if they all somehow took, then you'd have quadruplets, which wouldn't be viable. Five, then you could do a pickup. So I was hoping there was going to be enough to pick up or enough just to have sex, but not in the middle because then it's game over."

When Round Four produced two large follicles, the doctors told them to, wink wink, go book a hotel. The couple had been staying at Rae's stepfather's house whenever they were in São Paulo but during these precious, OB-sanctioned windows for intercourse, they made other arrangements—for everyone's sake. When they got the green light this time, they booked a room at a spot they'd dubbed the "Patrick Sex Hotel," since it was the place where they'd last conceived. After enjoying a few nights there, they took the usual redeye back to New York.

They had developed a friendly relationship with the ladies at the blood draw lab close to Rae's mom's place. They would come every two to three months to check HCG levels and always paid out of pocket because Rae wasn't insured in the US. They specifically waited until six weeks to test, afraid the numbers would be discouragingly low if they went any earlier. Previously her HCG had only risen to 100-150 mIU/ml, so when her levels tested over 4000 mIU/ml this time, the mood was celebratory.

They flew back to Brazil at around eight and a half weeks and scheduled their first ultrasound for the day they landed. They were disheartened to see an empty sac, but her HCG was still high. Because they'd had sex, not done a transfer, they didn't know the exact age of the embryo. The doctors said it was too early to tell.

This was the first time they'd ever gotten so far, and Rae hadn't expected to see a heartbeat. But it was a long week of waiting, half expecting the first signs of miscarriage but fully hoping this would be their lucky draw.

"Every round I thought I felt something," Rae explained. "Part of what was so nice about having Colin with me through this whole journey was checking, 'How crazy do I sound now compared to last month?' or 'I feel like my boobs hurt. Did I feel like my boobs hurt then?'" Rae nodded toward the desk. "This is the IVF notebook we started in October 2016."

"I was the keeper of the notebook," Colin announced, perking up. "For Raeanne, her way of dealing with uncertainty is researching and learning as much as she can, which isn't really my style." He shifted in his chair. "It just doesn't make me feel better. So my job was to write everything down so she could ask me questions later."

Colin also did the fertility-medication injections. Rae couldn't so much as look at the needles without squirming.

When Rae and Colin went back to the doctor the following week, they saw a fetal pole—a thickening on the margin of the yolk sac—but no heartbeat. The fetus was clearly growing but was noticeably underdeveloped for ten weeks. They were told to return again in a week. At that point, they were fairly sure a baby wasn't happening, but it was hard not to harbor any hope given the pole sighting.

It was another two weeks before the doctors pronounced the pregnancy unviable. At first, they hoped Rae's body would get rid of it on its own, but her HCG was holding steady. They tried to schedule her for manual aspiration or a D&C, but Rae refused. She just wanted it to be over already, so they could go hide out in Europe and forget about IVF for a while. In fact, she'd already booked flights for a month out so she'd have something to look forward to.

Rae was so desperate to avoid the surgery, she pleaded with her mother in Ohio to smuggle a dose of RU-486, the so-called "abortion pill" generally considered safe to terminate pregnancies up to ten weeks gestation, to her in Brazil. Rae figured the fetus had only developed to about six and a half weeks, although technically she was at twelve.

Her mother was hesitant. Not only would she be compromising her ethics as a doctor filling a dummy prescription for her daughter, but abortion was illegal in Brazil. There could be real consequences.

The couple couldn't say how the pill found its way to Brazil, but it did, and Rae took it immediately. As soon as she started bleeding, she felt the immense relief that the experience would soon be behind her. But it was still a shock.

"I couldn't stop thinking of it as baby material," she said with a wince.

She went through waves of contractions, followed by a rush of matter from her body. She felt uncomfortable about soiling herself or the mattress she was lying on, so she'd make for the bathroom whenever she felt the onset of cramps. One time she didn't make it to the toilet, however, and her body burst like a dam onto the bathroom floor.

"Have you ever seen calf's liver?" Rae asked, laughing. It's apparently one of her favorite foods, especially when she's pregnant. She made a sphere with her hands spread wide, fingertips barely touching. "This big. Grocery store–sized. Solid. That was the piece of tissue that fell on the floor."

Sobbing amidst what looked like a murder scene, Rae called for Colin. "I can't touch it," she told him. "I can't pick it up. I can't clean it. Please!"

Colin ran in with a roll of paper towels and wiped the room clean. "It was so bright red, it looked like someone had been decapitated," he recalled.

As Rae continued to bleed heavily well after the contractions subsided, her doctors worried about anemia. When they examined her, they found there was still a significant amount of tissue in the womb. They didn't think there was much left to clear so they suggested a manual aspiration, which wouldn't require fussy meds or a trip to the hospital.

Rae's all-male medical team—loud-mouthed, stubbornly macho Brazilian men—insisted that she should avoid a full-on D&C at the hospital. The aspiration would barely hurt and be over before she knew it, they told her.

Colin kept to the sidelines, encouraging Rae to do what she felt was right.

She agreed to aspiration—but the moment she arrived for the procedure, she regretted letting them talk her into it.

"It's a vacuum," she said flatly. "No anesthesia. Like, does someone have a valium? Nothing. Can I have something local? Nothing. They told me it would be quick . . ." She sighed and fell back in her chair, exhausted. "It was the worst of the worst."

A friend of hers later described manual aspiration as ten times worse than labor: "At least labor felt natural, whereas this was just wrong."

And to make matters worse, the procedure didn't clear out all the fetal tissue.

Rae was livid.

"A lot of my anger actually came out around that pill. Like, how hard is it to give yourself a fucking abortion?" Rae's eyes were wild. "I was so mad at everybody—the doctors, the providers, how long it was taking to terminate this thing, the whole process."

Colin nodded, biting his lip.

"I finally *get* pregnant, now I can't get *un*-pregnant!"

Rae needed the D&C after all—which, in retrospect, she wished she'd done from the outset. Getting rid of the pregnancy took a month longer than expected. Rae and Colin's flight to Europe, which they'd already had to reshuffle, was just days after the D&C. Rae was still bleeding when she boarded the plane.

Once Rae and Colin settled into a more of a relaxed holiday vibe in Europe, Colin realized he didn't want to go back to Brazil. He didn't want any more roundtrip tickets. He wanted off the IVF train.

"As a support person," Colin explained, "you're not only gearing up for your life to be transformed, you're going to battle. You're always on the cusp of this enormous thing—but then it doesn't come. So am I gearing up for this unfathomable amount of change or continuing my life as it is?"

The inertia was obvious, compelling, romantic—and exhausting. Colin desperately wanted a moment to take it all in and reevaluate their path to parenthood. It was a moment of reckoning. Until then, they'd always learned something new, something different to try the following round. They hadn't been processing the events of the past few years as losses of life but rather as years of banging their heads against a brick wall.

"There was always a next step, but after that last one, we didn't feel there was a next step," Rae said. "So it was a tough trip, although much needed."

Inertia won out; they returned to São Paulo after their trip, geared up for their fifth round of IVF. Then the letdown of a canceled transfer brought them back to New York for recovery.

The next trip to Brazil would be their last go at IVF.

Their final round was a success. To their immense joy and relief, they soon learned that twins were on the way.

I spoke with the couple a few weeks shy of their due date. Rae's grin was nearly as gigantic as her belly.

It wasn't until she was well into this pregnancy, she told me, that she began to process her losses—finally let her guard down enough to sit with her grief and acknowledge the difficulty of their journey.

She was glad she'd recently decided to get back on Instagram, where she'd quickly established supportive friendships with other women expecting twins, mostly via IVF.

Talking about her IVF struggles with others earlier on in their journey has helped Rae reflect on everything she and Colin went through. Sharing stories, she feels, is as cathartic for the listener—or "mentor," as Colin likened her—as it is for the storyteller. She regrets not divulging her own story sooner.

I wanted to know what else Rae thought might have supported her along the way. She paused to look at her husband.

"No one ever said to me, 'You'll probably do infertility treatments for the next five years and then just give up.'" She leaned forward with a serious look. "I would have loved to meet a forty-five-year-old woman who was like, 'Oh yeah, I tried and it didn't work, but I have a happy, fulfilling marriage; we just didn't end up having kids.'"

Rae had needed to hear that it would be okay if they weren't successful. That her whole world wouldn't collapse.

"Wouldn't that be an amazing story?" She threw her hands in the air. "Though I can't imagine anyone else dealing with infertility would want to hear it." She paused for dramatic effect. "But I would have! That's way more comforting than all the stories of someone's cousin who tried for six years then spontaneously got pregnant on vacation at forty-two. Not helpful!"

Was the blanket encouragement Rae heard during her IVF travails too artificial, too sunnily spun, to offer reassurance or encouragement to keep trying? I grappled with her paradoxical remarks—the tension between what we want to hear versus what we need to hear to find healing and support. If we recognize the potential value in something for ourselves, surely others would too, right?

Would I be one of those fortysomethings who finds peace and fulfillment without kids?

Rae leafed through the notebook, emitting sighs and the

occasional giggle. "Look! Up until we got pregnant, and now there aren't any pages left." She was radiant.

The last entry was from February 13, 2019, the day before our call. I asked if she wouldn't mind reading it.

"Thirty-six weeks, five days, went to the lab," she read.

Colin looked on like a proud father.

"Big tests. Heartbeats of the babies look good. Baby one: 46cm, 3.0 kilos. Baby two: 45cm, 2.8 kilos."

Two weeks later, Rae messaged me photos of the twins. She had just returned home to their new apartment in São Paulo after recovering from a complicated C-section. The last four years had been grueling, and the final stretch had been no exception. Yet there they were on my phone, the literal fruits of her journey: two plump nuggets with Rae's beige complexion and thick, dark hair.

Caio and Rafaela's parents had, at last, found their happy place.

CHAPTER 8

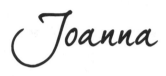

"I knew my babies were out there."

FROM HER ROSY APPLE CHEEKS to the disarming way she invited me into her homey California kitchen for tea, Joanna radiated motherly vibes. Holiday cards with cheery family faces and costumed pets adorned the fridge and overflowed onto the molding in the dining room, where we sat at a wood butterfly table half-bedecked in mail and laundry. As we tested the mic and recording levels, I noticed something familiar about Joanna that transported me to my childhood.

"You've got quite the radio voice," I observed.

"Really?" Joanna's brow lifted. A curly blond bob framed her round, smiling face and distinctly flat nose.

"My parents worked in radio," I explained, tapping my fingers on the table, suddenly sheepish about my comment. "My earliest years were a soundscape of DJs, producers, and Top 40 hits."

"Oh yeah? Funny." She nodded with a light chuckle. "Before my boys were born, I used to produce commercials."

I relaxed with the knowledge both that my intuition wasn't completely off and that Joanna's story didn't end in the dramatic loss for which she'd primed me. There were multiple children.

"Now I do two or three part-time gigs so I can be available for them."

Joanna, in her early fifties, knew from the time she was six years old that she wanted children. Marriage, she could take or leave. Both her parents had divorced several times, so she didn't have a particularly optimistic view of the institution.

"Having children was this obvious, forgone conclusion." Joanna's lips glided into a smirk. "For no good reason, I always assumed it would be easy to get pregnant."

Though Joanna had dated men for years and was far from vigilant about using protection, she never got pregnant. When she began seeing women, in her early thirties, the realization sank in that there might be obstacles to conceiving, so she researched what it would take to create a family with a woman. She joined a group of local lesbians figuring out their path to motherhood, where she gained valuable tips from many women who would become lifelong allies.

Joanna found herself single at thirty-seven, which she described as "one of those ages commonly referred to as your fertility dropping off a cliff as you stand there, the earth crumbling beneath you." With the help of her longtime therapist, Joanna came to understand that she was not prepared to have a child on her own, despite an increasingly urgent desire to procreate.

"People who choose to single-parent? More power to them!" she said with a tap on the table. "Honestly, the life partner aspect was secondary for me. I needed a partner who wanted children."

Two years later, Joanna met Tamara, then forty-seven. On their second date, unsure where things were headed, Tamara asked, "So, do you want kids?"

Joanna pounced. "Absolutely! You?"

"Nope, not me," Tamara replied smugly.

Joanna figured there wouldn't be a third date—but the chemistry was too strong to keep them apart.

As things got more serious, the issue eventually came to a head. While Joanna felt gun-shy about committed relationships because of her parents' collective eight marriages, her partner was even more dubious. Tamara's father had been killed when she was three, and her mother had remarried ten times. Still, for Joanna, having children was paramount.

"I can't imagine my life without children," she told Tamara.

"I can't imagine *your* life without children," Tamara said, taking her hand. "I get it."

"I wanna be clear," Joanna leveled with her. "I am not looking for support as I parent a child; I'm looking for a life partner *and* my parent partner." She paused for a deep breath. "Are you in?"

"Babe, I'm terrified." Tamara squeezed Joanna's hand. "But . . . I'm willing to have a child with you . . . just this once!"

They smiled at each other through tears.

"Well . . . okay!" Joanna said. "Yes!"

Joanna let out a big belly laugh as she recalled the scene, her eyes ablaze with adoration for her wife.

At the time, Joanna thought thirty-nine was old to try to conceive, but that things would work out. She'd get inseminated and have their child, and life would go on.

"I grieved a little because I never wanted to have just one child," Joanna confessed. "Being an only child would be hard . . ." She paused, searching for the right word. "Sad." Joanna and Tamara had over a handful of siblings each. "How lonely it would be, and then that child grows up so quickly surrounded only by adults."

I nodded, feeling grateful for my two older brothers, who heavily shaped the woman I've become.

Joanna transformed the disappointment of not having a big family into the focused fervor of getting pregnant. She used the word "we" to describe most of the steps to achieving this end; though it was her body, the mothering journey was something she and Tamara did together.

The most logical place to start was IUI. Joanna and Tamara picked out sperm like some mothers might scrutinize their child's fiancé—was he intelligent, attractive, healthy?

Once they chose their donor, Joanna did IUI half a dozen times, but nothing took.

"I was honestly shocked," she told me, shaking her head.

She poured herself into research on IUI challenges, including possible infertility, and had a host of tests done to narrow in on the problem. It seemed like one of her tubes might be blocked, but that was soon ruled out. The doctors couldn't say why she wasn't able to conceive.

"It's fascinating how little we 'regular women' know about pregnancy and infertility," I said.

"Oh, tell me about it!" Joanna sighed, smiling.

Joanna's response to both her doctors' and her own inconclusiveness—or ignorance, depending on her mood—was education.

"Head down, I immersed myself." Joanna cleared her throat. "Privately, of course, because I couldn't say anything at work."

In her highly competitive field, Joanna feared pushback from demanding clients, with their busy schedules, as well as the more ominous threat of demotion. She was putting in sixty-plus hours a week, with a lengthy commute across the Bay into San Francisco, and traveling every other month. She had to be prudent about scheduling her clinic visits and was careful not to mention anything about trying to conceive to anyone at work.

"I worked in a company with seventy people and didn't want to risk losing promotions," she explained. "Our projects were nine months to a year and a half, so why put me in a really good position if I couldn't finish the job?"

"Never mind discrimination laws," I joked.

"Right!" She laughed. "It was an odd contrast of being so excited yet unable to talk about it."

Outside of work, Joanna pulled in her entire community. "Okay," she told them, "here's what's going on. I need everyone's support, all the good vibes. You want to meditate every night or say your morning prayer for us? Great, we'll take it."

But the positive thoughts weren't enough to get Joanna pregnant.

After a year of IUI, just shy of her fortieth birthday, Joanna's doctors urged her to consider IVF, saying, "You've got no time to waste."

In anticipation, Joanna had been seeing a fertility acupuncturist for years. She'd exhausted all other options available, short of IVF, and had enough vials of sperm in reserve for several treatments.

After weighing the pros and cons, she and Tamara decided to dip into their savings and try a round of IVF.

On the first attempt, the couple was able to harvest a handful of successful follicles. Then they were faced with the question of how many to put into Joanna's womb.

"There I was, with this woman who was super clear on just wanting one child," Joanna said, raising her brow with a half-smile. "Well, we put in two knowing the odds of successful implantation from fresh IVF with frozen sperm was 18 to 20 percent."

Joanna beat the odds and got pregnant.

"I was over the moon!" she howled. "We both were, although Tamara was still freaked out. But, here we go! Life's beginning!" She pumped her fists victoriously. "This really had been one of my life goals, my vision, for so long."

Joanna was finally pregnant, but the couple still lived apart. Tamara was an hour's drive from Berkeley, in Sonoma. They spent weekends together, and Joanna scheduled her clinic visits in the city on the few days a week when Tamara also commuted to San Francisco.

"I made her come to every single appointment," Joanna told me. "I say 'made' because it wasn't an ask. I simply stated my expectation that we do it all together, and she agreed."

Around seven weeks gestation, alone in her apartment on a

late weeknight evening, Joanna noticed some spotting. They'd just seen a heartbeat earlier that week. She called Tamara, normally an early riser, for support, but Tamara never quite awakened to the conversation.

Joanna didn't want to blow things out of proportion, but the spotting soon became more consistent, so she called a nurses' hotline and booked herself an appointment for the next morning at her clinic. She wanted to call Tamara back and express the urgency she felt—"Wake up right this minute! You might need to drive down here!"—but she let her sleep.

When Joanna awoke to more bleeding, it took everything she had to call work and come up with a convincing lie so she could address the well-being of her future baby.

I asked what was going through her mind.

"It'll be fine. It'll be fine. It'll be fine." Joanna rocked slightly in her chair. "If I will it to be, it'll be fine."

Joanna arrived at the clinic with damp cheeks and a saturated menstrual pad. A nurse took a sample to check her HCG level.

"We can't tell," the nurse said when she returned later that hour, "but it seems you've miscarried."

Joanna's heart sank.

"Do you want us to do an ultrasound?" the nurse asked.

Joanna initially fretted over the additional expense, but her heart quickly won out. "Absolutely, I want an ultrasound!" she cried. "What does that cost?"

Joanna couldn't hear the nurse's reply over the racket in her head.

"Yes, please squeeze me in now," she heard herself saying.

Soon an ultrasound technician was tracing the contours of Joanna's belly.

"There's nothing there," the woman said softly.

Joanna wept on the exam table, holding her empty womb. "Can I just have a moment here?"

The technician left Joanna alone to get dressed. When the nurse returned, some confusion ensued.

"There's very little chance . . ." She paused. "We'll still run the numbers, though. What do you want to do next?"

Joanna couldn't make sense of the situation. All she could think was, *Back the fuck off.*

Through exasperated tears, she told me, "On the one hand, they were saying it's really clear, but on the other, there's a chance I might still be pregnant? Such a mixed message!"

She needed closure or hope—not both. She quickly pivoted to problem-solving mode; she knew she needed time to grieve, but not then and there. She wanted to know the logistics of getting pregnant again.

"We're paying storage on a frozen embryo that we went through a lot to get," Joanna said, then proceeded to rattle off her most pressing questions: "I assume now my body knows how to get pregnant, so how long is the waiting period to try again? Do I need a D&C? What about the embryos? How do I figure these pieces out?"

The clinicians responded patiently to each of Joanna's concerns. By the time she left, she had a plan. But she had to ask for their guidance every step of the way.

"I was not quietly grieving," Joanna recalled. "I was alone, so they couldn't give the information to someone shepherding me—though maybe that's my projection, they might deal with unaccompanied people all the time. But although I was a mess, I still felt capable. So lay it all out!" She boomed this out with a swipe of her hand above the table. "I was in go-mode."

"It sounds like that's who you are," I said.

"Yep! Head down, this is only a stumbling block. I'm having a baby, damn it. Let's just figure out how!"

Tamara drove down that afternoon to comfort Joanna, and they agreed the long distance had to end. They'd been planning to wait 'til further along in the pregnancy to find a home together.

New plan.

Acupuncture played an integral role in Joanna's recovery, both physically and emotionally. She found out years later that her acupuncturist had also miscarried—within days of Joanna. Although they were friendly before she was an acupuncturist, the woman hadn't mentioned the loss to Joanna because she felt that as her doctor, she should keep it private.

"That was really difficult," Joanna said, "and I told her what a disappointment it was."

"She was holding space for you," I suggested.

"Yes, but it would have helped me to know that someone else was going through it." Joanna looked up at the ceiling, steadying back tears. "If she had said, 'I totally get it, and I'm with you,' I would've felt *more* held, energetically."

Joanna's reflection stung; I'd intentionally gone out of my way to hide my miscarriage from coaching clients. By not being forthright about the nature of my canceled appointments, I realized, I may have squandered an opportunity to help someone in need of support. I never doubted hiding the loss, for fear of being seen as unprofessional. Now I questioned, as a coach, how well I practiced what I preached: *Show up as your whole self, the shadows and the light.*

Joanna, too, struggled with presenting her whole self.

"The balance of having room to grieve but also actively moving on was so hard—and all in private!" she cried. "I didn't have any shame about miscarrying. I didn't feel my body betrayed me. More than anything, I was thrown. Like, clearly I'm supposed to have a child, so why?"

Joanna has since talked to a number of women who say they remember the date of their miscarriage and mourn each anniversary. Not her.

"Honest to God, I have no idea what the date was. It's not something I carry closely," she said. "As painful as it was, there wasn't a damn thing I could do about the loss."

Once Joanna and Tamara had moved in together, the next major challenge was the financial reckoning with IVF.

"Babe, how can we afford to do this again?" Tamara paced the living room. "What are we doing here?"

"I don't know what the plan is," Joanna said quietly, looking stern, "or what I'm going to have to sell . . . but we have to keep trying."

"Right, but we just blew through $30,000, which we weren't exactly planning to spend. We could swing it the first time, but this is a big leap from IUI." Tamara gave her a pleading look. "Holy shit, Joanna, this is expensive!"

"Tam, we have a pretty comfortable lifestyle. Not amazing, but we can do this. We'll find a way."

Tamara joined Joanna on the couch and let out a long sigh. "Okay," she said as Joanna pulled her close. "I guess we'll figure it out."

Barbara, one of Joanna's close friends, had done eight fresh cycles of IVF before successfully giving birth to twins. In the throes of trying to conceive, Barbara had taken a job at the women's clothing chain Casual Corner, an hour and a half drive away, because she knew their health insurance plan would cover two IVF cycles. She encouraged Joanna to keep trying and trust that the money would work itself out.

Joanna did two more rounds of IVF, and neither one resulted in pregnancy. That year, she and Tamara claimed a whopping $104,000 in health expenditures on their tax returns.

After so many failed attempts to get and stay pregnant, Joanna briefly considered adoption, but in her heart she knew it wasn't for her. She had concerns about birth parents and losing one's kids. Friends of theirs who'd foster-adopted had gone through two years of potential reunification with the original family, only for their children to be taken away in the end. "I can get through anything, but I didn't want to put myself through that," Joanna said with a single nod of emphasis.

Plus, she wanted to experience the full range of motherhood—
pregnancy through delivery included—which was something that
adoption could not provide. She also viewed pregnancy as a natural
buffer to parenthood. "It's important we start being parents before
someone hands us a baby," she told me, laughing. "I also just really
wanted to be pregnant. That was always my vision."

My heart fluttered; Joanna was speaking to my deepest longing to
experience pregnancy—sore breasts, vomiting, and all.

Joanna remained undeterred by the financial and emotional set-
backs, but she and Tamara did have to confront the facts of their
situation: Joanna was forty-one now, and her window to carry a pregnancy to term was dwindling.

"I knew my babies were out there." Joanna stared at me hard. "I
just had to remove the obstacles between them and me."

Apparently, one of the obstacles was Joanna's eggs, so they would
need both sperm and egg donors—a complete embryo.

"I think of myself as a spiritual person, not religious," she said,
"but essentially that was my faith: my babies are out there."

After commiserating with an older friend who had previously
paid storage on seventy-five frozen embryos despite being over fifty
with two teenage children, it dawned on Joanna that there were likely
thousands of frozen embryos out there waiting for a match like her
and Tamara. They just needed to find the right donor.

The couple began shopping themselves around, asking everyone
they knew who'd done IVF for their leftover embryos. Joanna even
floated the possibility of her younger sister donating her eggs, but the
timing wasn't right.

Growing more desperate by the day, Joanna created a flyer with
color photos of her and Tamara and left it in her acupuncturist's office.

"I can't believe I did that!" she cackled. "I just thought, *Screw it, I
don't want this to be a secret*—I mean, I still wasn't out at work, but I
could keep that separate."

Joanna's mother, who lived in Albuquerque, suggested that she speak with someone at the free weekly there to see if they'd run a story on her. "It can only put energy in the right direction," she told Joanna.

With Joanna's permission, her mother tracked down a cub reporter, and soon enough Joanna was on a phone interview about the challenges of fertility. "It was so far outside my comfort zone, I couldn't even see my comfort zone!" she recalled.

When Joanna searched online, nearly all the organizations matching embryo donors with families were religious. *There's no way they'd want to give embryos to a lesbian couple*, she thought. This was less than fifteen years ago, but even liberal California has come a long way since then. "Knowing discrimination against gays was so pervasive—at least back then—was really discouraging," she said.

Eventually, she stumbled upon Miracles Waiting, a nondenominational site. "No religious fluff," Joanna said, "just a nonprofit founded by people who had gone through it and wanted to help people connect."

It was 11:00 p.m. the night she found Miracles Waiting, and Joanna had to be up at 4:30 a.m.

"I didn't care about sleep. I was immediately sucked into a vortex reading all the ads," she said, laughing. It felt like a long shot, given how targeted the ads were, but somehow more manageable, more promising, than an article in the free weekly in Albuquerque or the many faith-based organizations that required home visits prior to sanctioning embryo donations.

By midnight, Joanna had started answering ads and posted her own listing for $75.

Joanna was out with a friend when her phone lit up with a response to her ad.

"I completely lost it, sobbing in public." Her voice cracked. "So, I was right. Someone will find our family, the right match will find us. Not everyone will be judgmental because we're two California lesbians."

Two respondents contacted Joanna, who then diligently and covertly pursued both options: a single woman in Virginia with two children who'd chosen sperm based on the donors' success and intelligence, and a local lesbian couple with a son whose sperm-donor father was a close family friend. The latter didn't seem like "their people" but did seem compelling enough to explore. Both donors wanted an ongoing relationship with the future baby.

Joanna and Tamara were tasked with choosing the "right" embryo. There would soon be a mountain of documents to sign, and they worried about potential missteps in this legal grey area. Though they sought legal advice before signing with both parties, Joanna agonized over the decision.

"The soul of our child will come through whichever embryo gets you pregnant," Tamara reassured her. "When we trip onto the right path, our baby will be there."

They opted for the woman in Virginia and stalled with the local couple. After months of discussions, more legal documents, and complex shipping arrangements, it was finally time for the IVF transfer.

The doctor helped them choose the highest-ranked embryo of the Virginian's bunch and they went ahead with the transfer.

Much to everyone's dismay, Joanna's womb didn't take to it.

Heartbreak and regret spiraled into an anxious cacophony in Joanna's mind. She doubted her stubbornness. Was she wrong about her path? She was scared and careening toward forty-three. This was the first time she'd allowed herself to think about the possibility of her pregnancy plans not panning out.

I was so caught up in her story, I glanced nervously around the room, searching for some sign of validation that Joanna indeed had children. When my eyes landed on a photo of two flaxen-haired boys resembling the woman across from me, a sigh escaped my lips, barely audible over Joanna's hearty voice. But were those boys hers?

Ever determined, Joanna pushed past the temporary defeat and forged ahead with the local couple's donation. She had the three donated embryos transferred in a single cycle of IVF, introducing the small but real risk of triplets and the ensuing danger of miscarriage for any or all of the fetuses that might develop. If Joanna became pregnant with all three, she would be faced with the impossible decision of having to "deselect"—effectively, abort—one of them, as carrying three to term would be medically inadvisable. Still, the odds were less than one in five that Joanna would get pregnant at all.

Following the transfer, Joanna tried everything she imagined might help: legs up, eating pineapple for a healthy uterine lining, regular acupuncture, recruiting her friends' and family's well wishes.

When bloating and fatigue set in, the first bud of hope bloomed.

Joanna's mother flew in to accompany Tamara and her to the first ultrasound visit at six weeks gestation. Nerves were running high when the doctor looked up from the screen. He met each woman's gaze as he burst into a smile, flashing two fingers in the air. Twins.

"Tamara was shell shocked!" Joanna slapped the table. "Literally nonverbal for five hours. Meanwhile, I'm"—Joanna bobbed her head wildly and gobbled like a turkey—"because the vision I'd been holding all along was that we'd have two. I. Was. Elated!"

Ever the supportive partner and excited mom-to-be, Tamara quickly embraced their good fortune. The couple joked that she'd said one *pregnancy*, not one child.

Joanna was still in her first trimester when her boss offered her the opportunity to produce her own show. Being the lead would require a fifteen- to eighteen-month commitment and frequent travel to Los Angeles for work with a major celebrity. Joanna had been there seven years—and it had been a great run—but her real life's work, raising a family, had finally begun. All along, Joanna had planned to get pregnant, take maternity leave, and never look back.

Screw it, she thought, *all my cards on the table.* She asked her boss's superior, Lori, if she had a moment to talk. It wasn't the time to dilly-dally with middle management—especially the cold-shouldered, younger man who was her direct boss.

Lori ushered her in with a wave of her hand. "What's up?"

"I'm pregnant," Joanna blurted out.

Lori screamed, and colleagues came rushing to the door to see if she was okay.

Joanna forged ahead, "With twins."

Lori squealed and stormed out from behind her desk to give Joanna a long, swaying hug.

As colleagues wandered back to their cubicles, the two women began plotting Joanna's exit strategy. "Only do what you can manage," Lori reassured her. "We'll have a new lead primed for when you need to leave. We're just thrilled to have you 'til then."

Joanna couldn't believe her good luck.

The pregnancy was all Joanna had hoped it would be—at once physically exhausting and exhilarating, deeply fulfilling, and medically successful. She gave birth to fraternal twins—the boys in the photo I noticed earlier, now age seven.

From conception through delivery and beyond, Joanna was grateful to have a female partner. She felt she and Tamara had a leg up on heterosexual couples struggling with infertility.

"For straight women who don't anticipate any obstacles, it takes far more effort and resilience to get to where Tam and I started," Joanna said. "We knew it wasn't just going to happen, like so many straight people assume. I had to be proactive—researching, finding support, knowing not to feel guilty."

While Joanna described her wife as "really supportive but sort of blissfully ignorant," she knew that Tamara could relate by virtue of sharing both the female psyche and anatomy.

"If I'd been with a man, no matter how supportive he was, he doesn't have the same stuff." Joanna gestured to her breasts and pelvis. "He couldn't be supportive from a place of viscerally understanding cycles and a woman's body. That was a real advantage of being with a woman."

Being queer came with the added perk of a certain familiarity with being different as well, Joanna explained. Joanna, Tamara, and their queer circle already understood what it was like to live outside the box, which may have helped Joanna move beyond the shame felt by so many women dealing with fertility issues.

I asked Joanna, "If you could wave a magic wand, what would you change about your experience of fertility and loss?"

"I don't know that I'd change a thing," she replied, her pensive, pursed lips dissolving into a smile. "It's shaped who I am today and given me two beautiful children."

Given her hard-fought wisdom, Joanna said she was considering becoming a fertility advocate. "I don't really know the right term— pre-birth coach, pre-birth doula, fertility coach?"

We had a good laugh about the ever-changing jargon of women's health.

"There's so much new and shifting information about fertility and pregnancy, and it's hard to find and make sense of it all. Especially if you're an emotional wreck, trying to navigate the grief and loss and uncertainty . . ." She waffled over whether the work would serve her, and if she could meaningfully serve others.

"I would absolutely want you in my corner!" I whooped.

Joanna smiled bashfully, then disappeared into the kitchen with a mother's pride to gather photos of her children.

CHAPTER 9

Noreen

"You just end up quiet."

WE WERE ONLY A FEW MINUTES into talking about miscarriage when Noreen accidentally knocked over her wine. Shards of glass covered the table, pinot noir spilled over its edge, and a startling amount of blood gushed from Noreen's fingertip.

She maintained an aura of stately calm amidst the flurry of waiters and hostesses scurrying about our table cleaning up. She thanked each one while pressing a napkin to her finger to stop the bleeding. Her relaxed elegance evoked for me a finishing school dropout who couldn't quite shake the charms she had learned. She wore a large diamond ring, a gold lavalier necklace, pearl stud earrings, and a beach-casual ensemble.

"I am cut, but I'm just going to live with it and be fine," she assured me with a light-hearted chuckle and gentle toss of her chestnut bob as a waitress placed an open first-aid kit in front of Noreen as if it were a plated meal. "I'm used to crises. Can you tell?"

It had been over twenty-five years since the last of Noreen's three miscarriages, and the subject still made her jittery.

"It certainly brings out emotions," she confessed, leaning in and rolling her eyes. "Though I healed so many years ago." Wrapping her finger in a bandage, she explained, "When I had Meghan, I swear it didn't affect me anymore. It was like, this is right. This is the beauty of life."

Noreen, sixty-six, owns a handful of boutique hotels on the California coast. She overtook operations after cancer struck her late husband, Tom. She has Meghan, twenty-four, whom she had with Tom, plus Tom's two older daughters from a previous marriage, Laura and Jolie. Noreen is now remarried, but all her pregnancies were with Tom.

When Tom and Noreen got together, she was far more focused on her administrative career than on starting a family. It wasn't even on her radar until Tom, in his typically charming manner, convinced her that she might miss out if they didn't have a baby of their own. He knew he had married a romantic, so he appealed directly to her heart. The way he saw it, he told her, another child would bring the family closer together. Plus, Noreen would have the full experience of motherhood, including birth.

Noreen had tried the pill back in college, but it was far stronger in the 1970s and she'd never come around to it, so they'd been using other forms of birth control. Once Tom had successfully made his case for having a baby, it was only a matter of months before she was pregnant.

Tom was traveling for work the night it happened. Noreen was thirty-five years old and eleven weeks along. She went into the bathroom during the night and was shocked to see blood all over the floor.

"It was really ugly," she told me, her long, sun-kissed hands waving about. "And the bathroom was quite large!" She laughed nervously, shifting in her chair.

Noreen filled the sink with warm soapy water, got on her hands and knees, and scrubbed the floor. With each scouring motion, her pelvis screamed with pain. She focused her attention on the task at hand, moving from one tile to the next, until the floor was immaculate. Then she threw on some sneakers and drove herself to urgent care.

She didn't want anyone to see the blood, not even her husband. "I'm not a private person, per se," she tried to explain.

As we kept talking, she wondered aloud if she had felt ashamed.

When she got to the hospital, staff notified her OB, who drove over immediately. He had Noreen call Tom to let him know what was going on, so she wouldn't feel like she was alone. It never occurred to her to reach out to anyone.

"I've always felt that I could manage my own life," she said.

I knew this about Noreen from our time together studying executive coaching some years ago. The training program required us to bare both our strengths and weaknesses so that, as coaches and leaders, we would be able to encourage others to do the same. Noreen's independence shone bright from day one.

Noreen stayed in the hospital overnight and the staff did a D&C the following morning. She would have preferred to get it over with right away, but that wasn't an option. Tom booked the first available flight back and met her at home that afternoon.

They didn't tell anyone about the miscarriage except for Laura and Jolie, both teenagers at the time. Noreen didn't think there was enough awareness or understanding about pregnancy loss to feel comfortable speaking openly about it. She assumed people wouldn't care or think that it mattered. Her own doctor had explained that the miscarriage was the body's way of purging a fetus that wasn't viable. She figured if doctors were so matter-of-fact about it, others might feel similarly.

"So where do you get any solace out there?" Noreen asked, shaking her head. "You just end up quiet." She paused and stared into her new glass, then took a sip.

She believes her extended family and friends would have been supportive had she told them. But she didn't. She was scared of all the wrong things people might say.

"I felt like, because of what the doctor said to me, that they would discount it too, say, 'Oh, you're so much better off,' or 'God's will'—things like that." Noreen gyrated in her chair, a constant swirl of motion, then froze. "I would've just freaked if they'd said that to me."

Noreen's family was practical. "It was meant to be" was just the sort of thing they would have said, and she felt sure it would send her over the edge—her feelings, if not her entire being, rendered meaningless. She worried that if they didn't respond with the compassion she was seeking, old wounds would resurface. Why risk that when she was already feeling so miserable?

That doctor's language about "purging" and viability still haunted Noreen. She found it so jarring that she eventually switched to a female ob-gyn.

On the brighter side, the experience did bring Tom and Noreen closer as a couple. It was an intimate pain and secret they shared, a challenge they would find their way through together.

I wondered how Tom had coped with the loss—if he was able to provide comfort for Noreen.

"He might not have been profusely crying, but he was cuddling and . . . you know . . ." She looked down at her hands. "He felt bad. I knew he felt bad."

Noreen discovered the importance of female friends. She learned from the miscarriage that she needed to protect herself from ever feeling that isolated again and knew that Tom wouldn't be able to give her all that support on his own. "Life was going to hit me with more hard knocks, and I didn't want to be without my girlfriends," she explained. She reconnected with several friends from college and has remained close with them since.

It took months for Noreen to recover physically. It was by far the most traumatic of the three miscarriages she would ultimately experience.

Noreen said the next few years, from the late 1980s until Meghan's birth in 1995, were a blur. The second and third miscarriages took the wind out of her sails. She was getting older, was now in her late thirties. Time was running out.

"It's a lot of pressure!" Noreen practically bounced out of her chair. "Women are taught that family's everything."

At first, I understood Noreen to be speaking from a bygone era—the feminist backlash of the 1980s, when she was trying to conceive, or even the socially conservative 1950s of her youth. Later, however, it became clear that she meant women are *still* conditioned to prioritize family and motherhood. While today they might enjoy more child-care support from their partners and employers, women continue to learn at a very young age that family is the very essence of life. The stigma against cisgender, heterosexual women who choose to be childfree has not lessened with time. The expectation and assumption that all women can and will have children persist.

I, too, felt that pressure. Would my family and friends really understand if they knew that we were content without kids? Would I still feel some underlying pressure five years from now, in my mid-forties, with the possibility of having kids still open?

Noreen and Tom found some relief in knowing that they already had a family. They would always have Laura and Jolie, even if Noreen wasn't able to have her own baby.

The details of the second miscarriage were a bit hazier, but Noreen did recall after the fact, "Oh, that was the plop-plop!"—the all-too-common experience of passing the fetal tissue as a clotted mass so dense you can hear it hit the bottom of the toilet bowl.

She had no recollection whatsoever of the third miscarriage.

"I must be really numb to that one," she said slowly, in a deeper voice, trudging through each word as if it were mud.

What she did remember was that the third loss brought a mounting sense of defeat. She and Tom weren't interested in going to a fertility clinic, let alone entertaining IVF. It wasn't about the money;

Noreen just felt that if it wasn't going to happen naturally, then it probably wasn't meant to be.

"We need to stop this roller coaster," Tom finally told her, and she agreed.

They decided it was time to move on with their lives—to embrace the idea of not having a child of their own.

The decision made to stop trying, Noreen threw herself back into work and her busy social life. She and Tom downsized from two homes to a small cottage and traded in their four-seater sedans for convertibles. They were pleasantly distracted and enjoying life.

Then, one evening, as they were standing together in their kitchen, Tom broke into a grin and gestured toward her chest like he was holding two melons. Noreen blushed with the dawning recognition that her breasts had become painfully sore. Pregnantly sore.

It turned out she was already a few months along. They were able to laugh off the premature car and home purchases and embrace their fertile fortune—thanks, in no small part, to their financial well-being.

"I was a nauseatingly happy pregnant," Noreen boasted. She relished her changing body and her growing connection with the magical creature in her womb.

I listened to Noreen in a state of intoxication, half glazed over, indulging my long-standing fantasy of experiencing all the wonders of pregnancy.

"Everybody experiences that bonding at some point, but through having a child, you become one person."

The bonding extended to Noreen's stepdaughters, who immediately fell in love with their baby sister. Tom's vision of bringing the family closer together had been realized.

"Love is energy," Noreen told me, her eyes intently focused, imploring me to listen closely. "By the time you deliver, you've had nine months of that energy. But when you bring a child into your life, how much energy are you willing to give? Because it isn't about the immediate love; that energy transforms into love and an eternal commitment."

Noreen and Tom had come full circle. In completing their family, they had weathered the loss and disappointment of previous miscarriages. Noreen began sharing their stories of loss and triumph with others who'd experienced pregnancy loss, and after hearing her open up so vulnerably to friends and colleagues, Tom became open to sharing his perspective too.

Noreen didn't think she knew anyone else who had miscarried when she experienced her first loss. Or if she did, nobody talked about it.

"I'm sure I'd heard the word before, but I didn't know anybody. I was caught off guard completely," she said, shaking her head like a pinball stuck between two flippers. "No knowledge."

Meghan's birth and the soothing salve of time allowed Noreen to gradually speak more freely. She became determined to be open about her miscarriages and let other women who'd miscarried know that they weren't alone.

Though the pain of those losses subsided long ago, Noreen still struggles to understand why they happened in the first place, and is frustrated that the medical world hasn't provided better answers for women. Practitioners might be more compassionate these days, she feels, but there still haven't been enough studies focused on understanding all the hows and the whys of miscarriage.

Noreen voiced being particularly struck by how many women still hold on to the misconception that they are somehow to blame for their loss. "Some women believe that they walked too far, or 'Oh, that physical exercise I did,' or 'Oh my god, we had sex, I shouldn't have done that!'" she said, lurching her head forward with each maddening example. "It's never going to be medically analyzed. You can analyze it socially and emotionally, but I don't think the medical world will ever put money into it." She paused for a sip of wine, then forced a smile. "I mean, how are they going to make money, right?"

This brought us to the sticky issue of aftercare, which Noreen's current husband was keen to weigh in on when he joined us for dinner after our one-on-one chat. Chris, an ophthalmological surgeon, saw the issue from the perspective of patient outcomes. The successful outcome for doctors treating pregnant women is a healthy baby, and aftercare for newborns and their mothers is clearly defined and well established. The unsuccessful outcome for doctors is pregnancy loss, for which there is no established protocol—particularly in the case of loss before twenty weeks—beyond ensuring that the mother's physical health is preserved.

Chris spoke confidently and with compassion for his fellow doctors, even as he seemed willing to expose their weaknesses and those of the healthcare system at large. Few doctors, he argued, care to dwell on a poor outcome, so they are disinclined to follow up with patients. Add the glaring financial disincentive to continue care when practitioners are already so pressed for time, and it is perhaps no wonder that such patients are underserved. Culturally and systemically, there will have to be major shifts if our healthcare system is going to start effectively addressing the needs of women who experience pregnancy loss.

I nodded to Chris in animated agreement, my mouth occupied with fish tacos, while Noreen lamented that things haven't changed much in the decades since her miscarriages. She was adamant that there ought to be more support groups and other aftercare services for women, especially those not as fortunate as she was.

"The support was missing then and it's still missing!" she exclaimed, nearly knocking over another glass of wine. "I've listened to too many women who go through it."

Her final words of wisdom on loss?

"It matters!" She pounded her fist on the table and looked me straight in the eye. "And don't let anyone tell you it doesn't!"

That evening, journaling on one of Noreen's hotel balconies overlooking the Pacific, I marveled at the strength she'd shown in overcoming the shame and stigma she'd felt around her miscarriages. She'd wanted to share her story not just with me but with as many women as we could possibly reach, so that they, too, could move beyond the shame—something so many of us who experience pregnancy loss still feel today, just as Noreen did over thirty years ago.

CHAPTER 10

Jackie

"I was entitled to feel a loss."

EMERSON KNEW FAR MORE about ovulation cycles than most eight-year-olds. Back when she was in kindergarten, the teacher went around the room asking what everyone's parents did for a living. She wasn't entirely wrong when she announced, "My mom's a nurse and Daddy makes babies." Her father Jonathan had been fully employed as an environmental engineer since before she was born.

Emerson's mother, Jackie, confided in her when she found out she was pregnant with Emerson's sister Althea. After so many miscarriages, friends and family had become desensitized to Jackie's grief, and she knew her secret would be safe with her daughter. Emerson was the oldest of two at the time, her brother Archie two years her junior. Before Althea was conceived, there were nearly four years of struggle, from fertility clinics to debilitating loss and depression. During that time, Emerson had become familiar with all things pregnancy-related. So when her mother showed her the test stick, she affirmed with a quick glance that it was positive. She said, "Mommy, you don't even have to take a picture of it; it's obvious," Jackie relayed to me proudly.

Jackie and I went to high school together in New Jersey. We hadn't spoken in twenty years when she messaged me about sharing her story. When we met again over Zoom, I saw the same big, blue eyes, fair skin, and dirty blond, shoulder-length 'do I remembered from the '90s. A venerable Amy Poehler, with slightly thinner lips and a remarkably similar, salty sense of humor.

The first few minutes of our exchange were interrupted by "Please get on the other side of the door, honey," and "Mommy needs privacy." It was a snow day in Maine, and everyone was home. "Apparently, having a meeting means nothing anymore," she said.

Jackie had her first miscarriage in freshman year of college. She was still dating her high school sweetheart, who, somewhere along the way, had turned abusive. Her parents had just gotten divorced. It was a challenging time for Jackie. In retrospect, she wondered if the loss may have been a blessing in disguise. The relief that she wouldn't have to make the decision herself was tempered by a hefty dose of Catholic guilt. Both she and her boyfriend had been raised in religious families. Abortion was not on the table. But the thought of being tied to that particular person at that particular moment was terrifying. She wanted a baby eventually—just not like that.

Once the miscarriage was over, she put it out of her mind. She had bought into the notion that everything happened for a reason. Ten years later, Emerson's birth affirmed that thinking.

"We were so passionately in love, so of course our love would create a baby," she told me with a broad smile.

Jackie, almost thirty at the time, was wrapping up nursing school in New Jersey, and Jonathan had just completed his master's and was working in Maine. They figured it was a good time to get pregnant. The long-distance issue was only temporary.

They were spending the weekend together in Mystic, Connecticut, about halfway between their respective homes, when they found out. Jackie woke up with a fierce hankering for oysters and was immediately intent on hunting down the best spot to enjoy them. While they walked along the cobblestone streets, admiring the old ships on the waterfront, she complained of a backache.

Jonathan, putting the pieces together, suggested, "Maybe you're pregnant."

"Nah," Jackie said, brushing it off. They'd only just started trying. *Nobody gets pregnant that quickly*, she told herself. "Go buy a test," she goaded him.

They went to the nearest drugstore and bought a pack of cigarettes and a pregnancy test.

"We must have looked super gross," Jackie explained to me, laughing. "But I really didn't think I was pregnant."

When they got back to the hotel, Jonathan asked Jackie to hold off doing the test until he came back from walking the dog. But Jackie couldn't hold it in, so she went ahead and peed on the stick and left it on the bathroom counter. When he returned, anticipating the excitement of the live test, she confessed the deed was done.

"You did it already?" he asked, his face falling into a frown.

"Jonathan, it's peeing on a stick. I couldn't wait!"

He pouted on the bed, averting her gaze.

"I can't believe you're being such a dick! God . . ." Jackie grabbed the stick from the bathroom and marched back in. "It's not even . . ." She looked down at the stick, then back at Jonathan. "Um. This is a positive test."

Jonathan shot up to see for himself, then threw his arms around her. They retraced the moment of conception and determined the baby couldn't be any bigger than a poppy seed.

Although he knew it was early, Jonathan wanted to go to Babies R Us right away and make a list of everything they were going to need. Jackie was skeptical at first but decided to indulge him.

"It was kind of exciting," she told me, "because it was the first time I was shopping for myself. I had been there a million times to buy shower presents for coworkers and friends. But then it was *me* planning what I wanted!" Her eyes widened and her shoulders bounced with the exhilarating memory. "Do I want giraffes? Do I want zebras? Yeah, I can get into this!"

Jackie's sister had announced her pregnancy two weeks earlier—instant cousins! Jonathan was obviously excited, so even though it was early, Jackie allowed herself to enjoy the moment as well.

When they were back in the car, Jonathan had a panic attack.

"He was hyperventilating and dry-heaving because he realized how much babies cost and had been doing this running inventory of the crib, the Pack 'n Play, the stroller—all the things! Where were we going to come up with the cash? I was in nursing school, so money was tight."

In the end, the finances came together and it was an easy pregnancy for Jackie.

"I just knew we were going to have a baby and this was it. Everything went off without a hitch. She was a giant, fat, ten-pound baby," she announced, her face aglow.

It reaffirmed what she had felt a decade earlier about not being ready. Jonathan was the partner she wanted to father her children.

When Emerson was eighteen months old, they decided they wanted another baby. Jackie and her sister were two years apart, and she felt that was a good pace. Ideally, they hoped for five kids.

They were only trying for a few months before Jackie was pregnant again.

Archie was a completely different pregnancy. Jackie suffered through gestational diabetes, preeclampsia, and a traumatic delivery. Archie ended up in the NICU for six weeks. With his cerebral palsy, he experienced significant developmental delays as a toddler. The family had to juggle physical and occupational therapy along with an overall high level of needs. It was a strain on Jackie and Jonathan's relationship.

"It was the worst year of our marriage by far. I think just for anybody, going from one to two kids—it's exponentially harder. Then having a special needs child and a child still in diapers, and you're away from any family or any kind of support system . . . It was a rough, dark year," she said with a practiced manner, her strained neck and arched eyebrows betraying the difficulty of that time.

Although they wanted to keep the momentum of growing the family, it took them until Archie was two-and-a-half and they had moved into a bigger house for them to feel ready.

After trying unsuccessfully for three months, they decided to see a fertility specialist. Jackie was nearly thirty-five, on the cusp of what's considered advanced maternal age. As with one in ten women of childbearing age[10], she had polycystic ovarian syndrome (PCOS), so the specialist prescribed Metformin to enhance her ovulation. The side effects were brutal—a host of gastrointestinal issues, nausea, mood swings—but they were committed to having another baby.

After months on the medication, Jackie finally got pregnant—then, at ten weeks, miscarried. They were devastated.

"Two years ago, it was just . . ." she sighed loudly. "I had Baby A, I had Baby B, so why now? I can make babies!" She looked up at the ceiling, steeped in her frustration.

Jackie fell into a deep depression. She had trouble focusing at work and it affected her performance. She stopped getting billable hours from her remote case-management office.

Jackie had always wanted a partner with a high emotional intelligence, but suddenly she felt like it had come back to bite her. Jonathan was as supportive as he could be, but it felt unfair that he wanted her to recognize his grief while she was actively mourning her loss. It wasn't going to work for both of them to be emotional and needy at the same time, especially not with two kids already demanding so much of their energy. If grief was going to be prioritized, then as the mother, shouldn't she grieve first? As a couple, they had to work through those tensions.

Jackie hadn't told anyone that she was pregnant. When she posted about the loss in her Facebook group of mostly moms, sharing how much harder it was than she had imagined, that she felt crushed and cheated by the miscarriage, the lack of support appalled her.

"I got some, 'Oh yeah, I've had miscarriages too,'" she told me, rolling her eyes, "but not in an 'I'm there for you, I know what it feels like' way."

The resounding message from friends and family was that her loss was insignificant because she already had two children. One friend tried to spin it positive: "Don't be sad, you already have two healthy kids!" Another offered, "Well, whatever the statistic is, it's only inevitable that at some point in your life you would have a miscarriage."

In her review at work that year, Jackie was pressured to account for the reduced hours and poor performance. She confided in her supervisor that she'd had a miscarriage. She disclosed her history of postpartum depression and said she was working through the grief. She apologized for letting her work get derailed but reassured her boss she was doing everything she could to get her head back in the game.

"I was honestly expecting some sort of report," Jackie told me. "As a nurse, I view miscarriage as a medical condition. Like, I *had* this and there's a medical reason why my behavior *is* this—but then she asked me if I was going to try for another baby!" Jackie practically flew out of her chair, her mouth agape. "Seriously! Are you *supposed* to ask that? It was very awkward . . . It turns out there was a whole culture there of No Children."

Within six weeks Jackie was fired, something she'd never experienced before (and hasn't since). She spoke with a lawyer friend who advised her that while workplace discrimination against women "happens all the time," it's incredibly hard to prove. Legally, a supervisor asking about an employee's intentions to get pregnant was overstepping—particularly in Jackie's case, where postpartum depression had negatively impacted her work. However, the burden of proof, not to mention legal fees, felt too great to bear. For someone already struggling with grief and depression, waging an uphill legal battle was not the path Jackie was prepared to take.

"It just added to all the other shit," she said, sinking back into her chair. "As if things weren't bad enough!"

Jackie went on to have two more miscarriages over the next year.

"As soon as we got the 'all clear' to try again, they changed my fertility medication," Jackie complained. "We had a hysteroscopy, did genetic testing, got my progesterone levels drawn—the whole nine yards! Everything looked fine. There was never any indication it wouldn't be a viable pregnancy. Until it wasn't."

Jackie switched doctors; her physician had left for a specialty residency and "was kind of an a-hole," she said. "I don't even know if he ever made eye contact; he was always at the computer or looking in the chart."

I asked Jackie if he also did her physical exams. "The guy who uses a speculum on you, right?"

"Yup. Personality of a dead fish," she said flatly. "As a healthcare provider, I don't need you to be my friend, I just need you to be good at your job. I wasn't expecting him to be super interested in my life, but having the recurrent miscarriages was emotional. If you can't do it yourself, send in a nurse or somebody who can be more sympathetic," she said, showing her true colors as a nurse. "Especially if you're going to be an Ob/Gyn, you *have* to be better prepared to give somebody bad news." Jackie wondered if her doctor sensed she didn't need all the pleasantries. "Maybe half of my mind *did* just want the facts, but half of me wanted somebody who was going to at least make the attempt to hold my hand," she said, those expressive eyebrows inching further up her forehead.

A friend who had struggled with infertility recommended a reproductive endocrinologist in Portland, about an hour drive from her home. When Jackie visited him, his support felt refreshingly authentic. While he respected her nursing credentials and didn't mince words, he treated her with real compassion.

The endocrinologist gave Jackie a prescription for Letrozole that her previous doctor had denied her because of its off-label use for fertility. She did Letrozole for ten cycles and ovulated on eight of them.

"If you're trying to conceive, you do five million pregnancy tests and you chart," Jackie said matter-of-factly. She became obsessed with charting her ovulation and pregnancies. She bought the tests in bulk on Amazon and peed on a stick once a day. She took pictures with her phone, then played with the photo filters to see if she could discern more conclusive results. "I'd swear I'd see something, but it wasn't always so clear. I would find out I was pregnant before most women would ever have a clue because I *wanted* to be pregnant. And I was a nurse," she added with a wink.

Jackie was ten weeks along when she lost the next pregnancy. Her blood work, including progesterone and HCG levels, had looked fine. Doctors couldn't explain why it had happened. She could only do so many cycles of Letrozole before it was medically advised to take a break or find an alternative. The pressure was on. Her doctor upped the dose, since she'd had a couple of cycles without ovulating, and after two more rounds she was pregnant again. With her furious charting, she knew very early on. But that knowledge wasn't enough to prevent another miscarriage, this time at six weeks.

"That's when shit got real," Jackie said, looking off to the side. "Still no reason why . . . My husband's four years older than I am, so if I didn't have a baby soon, that was it. We were never going to have a baby."

If Jackie didn't get pregnant in the last round of Letrozole, the next option was IVF. That meant a referral to the Boston IVF clinic and initial costs of $15,000. The couple could have pulled the money from their 401k, but they decided against the treatment.

"I had this immense guilt about borrowing against our retirement when we didn't even have college funds," Jackie explained.

Every month they didn't get pregnant and their youngest, Archie, became more independent, Jonathan harbored more doubts about growing the family. Did he really want to jump back into bottles and diapers and sleepless nights?

Jackie couldn't relate.

"I just didn't feel my family was complete," she said, her face reddening. "After the second miscarriage, people told me to take it as a sign, and was I 'really still trying?'"

Because I initially isolated myself after my loss, I didn't experience the disappointment of reaching out to my community only to be dismissed by those whose support I would have expected. I asked how Jackie processed those remarks and coped without the emotional support she'd anticipated.

"They're all moms, so they're super busy and lacking in their own self-care," Jackie explained. "They don't have a lot to give you. And then falling back to, 'But you already have a baby. Why does losing this baby hurt? People without children are suffering more than you.'" She was on a tear. "Well, who hurts more, and what's the appropriate level of depression and mourning I'm supposed to feel?"

She rejected the understanding of loss as relative. She spoke of her disdain for the term "rainbow baby," the child born after the metaphoric storm of miscarriage or stillbirth. In this parlance of loss, a "sunshine baby" was the child born before a loss; the child lost, an "angel baby."

"At what point are they no longer rainbows? How many rainbows are there? They're all rainbows, every child!" she cried. "I enjoy the ones that I have, and I still mourn the ones I don't."

Jackie often thought about the babies who didn't make it to term—how old they'd be, their personalities and influences in the family. It was a fine line to walk: paying respect to and acknowledging the losses without risking sliding into clinical depression over them.

"The 'rainbow baby' thing is a reminder of the loss," she said, "and I try not to dwell on it."

I asked if she was able to self-soothe or find support beyond her husband and friends.

"I get it where I can, but it's never really going to be consistent. Our lives are too chaotic," she explained with a wave of her hand. It was hard for Jackie to carve out her own time and not feel guilty about it. She was too focused on making a baby to think about herself.

"I'm a control freak," she said. "To not have control over getting and staying pregnant . . . There's no, 'Oh, you eat this' or 'You do this' or 'Put your legs up over your . . .' Nothing. There's no guarantee. So a huge source of my stress was having to surrender."

I asked Jackie how that affected her sense of womanhood. I knew my fertility challenges had distorted how I saw myself as a woman, and I still struggled to reconcile my understanding of womanhood divorced from being a mother.

Jackie paused, pursing her lips, and exhaled audibly through her nose.

"Our bodies are designed to do this. The idea that I did something to my body to cause this—I believed that myth. Was this punishment because I didn't take it seriously enough? Was the universe coming back to haunt me because there's some lesson here for me to learn?" She slouched and sighed, her eyes unfocused. Then she perked up and rapid-fire mocked her old self with a series of eye rolls. "All those years you should've been making babies but selfishly chose to get a degree! You only have so many eggs! Look, now you're advanced maternal age! Oh well, you get what you deserve!'"

Jackie recognized that the pressure to grow her family was largely internal. Deep down, she knew her expectations of herself were unreasonable.

"I viewed the losses as failures and the misconceptions as failures, so I felt like a double failure. Not only was I not conceiving, but then even when I did conceive, it wasn't viable."

To everyone's relief, Jackie got a break during that final round of Letrozole. With her daughter Emerson's early support keeping Althea's pregnancy a secret, Jackie eventually made it past all the big prenatal milestones and celebrated the baby girl's timely arrival.

Jackie knew it was over for having more children of her own, but she and Jonathan still wanted to grow the family beyond their three children, so they attended classes to become foster parents and have had several successful placements, from toddlers up to adults. With a license to host three placements at a time, they have always managed to accommodate everyone in their modest suburban home.

I still wanted to know how Jackie felt about the support she received from the medical community around the miscarriages. Could they have done more?

"There are other practices, like oncology, that have licensed clinical social workers available to talk to patients. So why not have a liaison available to talk to women about pregnancy loss?" she asked. "People who have to deal with stillborns or infertility, people who find out that they're never going to have children, people who have gynecological cancers—there should be somebody available in the office, without a referral, who can come in. I don't see why it's not in gynecology."

My recollection of Jackie as a fiery feminist prompted me to inquire, "Do you think it has anything to do with gynecology being solely about serving women?"

"For a lot of it, yeah!" She snickered. "You know, 'Women have babies in rice paddies! Your body is strong!'" she mocked. "All my babies were C-sections. I would have died if I'd had my ten-pound baby a hundred years ago."

While the medical world has made huge strides for women's physical reproductive health, she said, the mental health piece remains severely lacking.

I asked her what she would want to share with someone experiencing pregnancy loss.

"A lot of times I was harder on myself because I thought there were 'right' feelings," she reflected. "But I was entitled to feel a loss even though I have living children. My loss was just as valid. It shouldn't be second class." She shrugged. "People never know what to say when you have a loss, and 99 percent of the time it's the wrong thing."

I wondered if Jackie had any advice for people who mean well but struggle to express their support.

"In nursing school, one of the things we learned in therapeutic communication was if it's a really bad situation, you don't say anything. Don't try 'Oh, I've been through something similar.' Nobody who's going through hell wants to hear it. Your brain is in trauma mode, you're not ready to make those connections."

From a nursing perspective, the caregiver or friend should simply acknowledge the loss; "This is really difficult for you" or "I'm sorry, this is awful news" would be appropriate. Then the person can give space and see where things go from there, if anywhere.

It's not about forcing the conversation or putting a positive spin on it, Jackie said. "People will relativize it—'Well, it's good because you could have ended up with a baby with a chromosome defect,' or 'You could have been further along and that would've been so much harder.'" Jackie's grimace curled into a smile. "All of those situations suck! None of them is less sucky than the other!"

With certain wannabe supporters, Jackie decided it wasn't worth the effort; better to avoid the subject. Her sister, for instance, clearly felt enormous pressure to be there for her but constantly fumbled when trying to express her support. "It was almost a kindness not to have to put her in the position to be supportive," Jackie said, laughing.

Another coping tip of Jackie's that helped her through the worst of it?

Humor.

CHAPTER 11

Beth

"I needed to believe there was a greater purpose."

"I CAME TO SEE THE LIGHT," Beth said in her melodic drawl. "It was right around the holidays. Having kids biologically is not the only way to have kids."

That Christmas was the first without her grandmother, who passed away from cancer. She was especially close with Beth and, like most in Louisville, a huge college basketball fan. She and Beth used to joke that if she ever wanted to send Beth a message from heaven, she'd appear as a red cardinal, the University of Louisville mascot.

On Christmas Eve, Beth dreamt her grandma was floating toward her with bright red hair and a peaceful look. She never spoke, but when Beth asked her if she was pregnant, her smile grew. "Is it a girl?" she asked, and her grandmother's smile grew wider. She pressed a note into Beth's hand that read, *Great-grandma can't wait to meet your little one.*

When she woke up on Christmas morning, Beth rolled over to her husband.

"We're pregnant," she whispered.

"Really?" he asked, suddenly awake. "Did you take a test?"

"Nope—Grandma just told me," she said beaming.

When Beth took a test that day, it was positive.

The news was a blessing, and her grandma's gift couldn't have come at a better time.

"We were so excited, we wrote a poem and gave it to everybody gathered 'round the tree," she told me, giggling. "We kept it real close, just family."

When Beth was twelve, she was unofficially diagnosed with endometriosis, a painful disorder in which tissue similar to the uterine lining grows outside the uterus. An official diagnosis would have meant undergoing invasive procedures that could have compromised her ability to have children. Her symptoms were well understood in the family, as many female relatives suffered from it. Beth's mother had it too, and the doctors hadn't thought she'd ever have kids. After she had Beth, the miracle child, she had to have a full hysterectomy.

Because of her condition, Beth bled for twelve months straight; it was like a period that never ended and kept reminding her of its presence with constant cramping and stained clothes. When she was in seventh grade, her mom drove her to a mixer in town, and she bled so much between the time she stepped into the car and the moment she arrived at the event that she ruined the car seat.

"As if being a teenager wasn't hard enough," she said.

"That sounds awful," I muttered, thinking of several friends who had the disorder. I had no idea the extent of the horrors they must have gone through.

"Well," Beth said, with that Kentucky bounce in her voice, "it's just part of my tapestry and something that made me who I am today."

Even as a young teenager, Beth was concerned about her chances at motherhood.

After her initiatory year of symptoms, she was put on birth control to regulate the bleeding, an act that directly violated her religious beliefs.

"In family life class, the teacher made it crystal clear that birth control was against our beliefs," she told me. "But here it was, the only thing saving my life!"

Beth grew up with a Catholic father and a mother who was a member of the Church of Christ. Beth had mixed feelings about some of the messages she heard at school. After learning about the evils of birth control in class, she went home and cried to her mother.

"What's wrong, honey?" her mother asked.

"Mom, is God mad at me for being on birth control?"

"My gosh! If he hates you, then he hates me too!" she said, stroking her daughter's back. "No, no, no, you're fine. These are medical reasons."

Hearing her mother's acceptance allowed Beth to open her mind. She was grateful that she was being brought up in a home of multiple faiths and outlooks.

Beth is now thirty-five and a devout Catholic. She met her husband, Jason, in college, and by the time graduation rolled around they were inseparable. They both knew they wanted to be parents. For Beth, it was baked into her psyche and her soul—she was made to be a mother. When they first started dating, she told Jason she wasn't sure if she'd be able to have children, and that if she did they might be kids with challenges.

"I will embrace whatever I'm supposed to have and you might have to as well," she told him. "Are you on board?"

Jason said yes.

With some trepidation, Beth went off the pill after she and Jason got married. After twelve years of being on the medication that had saved her life, she now had to come off it so she could build a new life with her husband.

It took her body some time to adjust to producing its own hormones again. After a while, trying to conceive started to feel more like a job than a romantic act. Around the nine-month mark, Beth was ready to give up. It wasn't fun anymore; this wasn't how it was supposed to be. Eventually she decided, or rather conceded, that they would have to adopt.

Until they found out she was pregnant that fateful Christmas morning.

Two weeks later, Beth went in for her first ultrasound. She was six to eight weeks along. Everything looked great at that checkup, but the next day she noticed some spotting. Her doctor assured her it was normal but asked her to come back for another exam.

The ultrasound technician identified the source of the bleeding. She explained in technical jargon that what they had seen the day before was no longer the case. The fetus had detached from the uterus, was now cut off from any source of nourishment. Still, they were able to hear a heartbeat, albeit an intermittent one.

Before leaving the exam room, the technician made additional remarks that failed to acknowledge the severity of the news. Beth had pushed the exact words out of her mind by the time we spoke, but she still felt their sting.

"She was horrible," she said with a snarl. "She had lost all emotion to what she was doing. There she was, showing people glimpses of life, but this was just a job to her. If she would've just held my hand or asked me if I'd had enough time or taken more pictures—something that would have honored the moment. It was the last time I saw my baby and that would have made it a more cherished experience."

A nurse showed Beth to a waiting room with other post-ultrasound patients. She was in tears over the news when a woman walked in bitching to her husband because she'd just found out they were having twins. She yelled at him for doing such an injustice to her, moaned about having to raise two children now.

Beth was quick to sympathize—"Having twins is hard, I'm not judging"— but it was heart-wrenching to hear someone rail against the very thing she wanted so badly and had just lost.

Her doctor, more attuned to Beth's trauma, lent a human touch to the medical experience of her loss. As she held Beth's hand, she explained that the heartbeat was only audible because the baby girl was actively dying. There was still some life in her, but she was on her way out.

"My faith is strong," Beth said, looking into her doctor's eyes. "I'm not going to write this off. Miracles can happen any time."

"I know, Beth. I have to tell you, though, I have not seen that happen here. But that doesn't mean it's not possible." The doctor put her arm around her. "The likelihood is you're losing your baby. Do you want a D&C? Or come back in a couple days, and we'll see what we can do?"

Beth wanted neither. She couldn't accept the loss; nor would she accept any of the pain medicine the nurse practitioner offered her as she left the office.

"I needed to feel it," she explained. "I know not everybody should have to feel it, but I needed to know for myself that it was real."

At home that night, the bleeding worsened.

"It was the most excruciating pain in my life," Beth recalled. "I was lying on the couch then crawling to the bathroom, because I didn't have the strength to walk."

Beth hadn't anticipated that it would be so bad. Jason was at work, so she was alone going through labor, as she later understood the experience.

Beth passed the fetus in the toilet. The moment she flushed it down, she twinged with regret.

"I didn't fully connect all the dots," she said. "It was horrific."

Beth crawled back to the couch and felt like she'd just hit the lowest point of her life. Her baby was gone, just like that, down the drain. What had she done? The pain was far worse than anything she'd experienced with endometriosis. She lay slumped over a pillow, doubting whether she would ever be able to carry a child to term.

The nurse practitioner called that evening to check in on her. Beth still declined to take any pain medicine.

When the call came, Beth was watching the Casey Anthony trial on TV—the 2008 case of a young Florida woman accused of killing her two-year-old daughter—and was consumed with anger. Life and death, heaven or hell—it all seemed so cruel and arbitrary. She was furious with God.

When Beth's aunt rang later that night, Jason told her she wasn't in the mood to chat. Her aunt persisted. She was the only family member Beth knew of who'd had a miscarriage, so she relented. Her voice was nearly shot from all the crying when she picked up the receiver.

"I've been thinking of you all day. I was mad that your grandma came to tell you this news only for it to be ripped away." Her aunt sighed. "But it hit me, darling, it hit me. What was on the note that your grandma gave you?"

"Great-grandma can't wait to meet your little one," Beth answered quietly.

"Don't you realize your baby wasn't meant to be here? Your grandma was gifting you with the knowledge that God needed her and she would be waiting for you. She was gifting you the faith to see that it was destined for something more."

It dawned on Beth that her faith was the only thing that would hold her together. She needed to believe that there was a greater purpose. Her aunt was right. This was the essence of what her grandma had been communicating to her.

She and Jason named their daughter Hope.

Three months later, Beth was pregnant with Jacob, who is now seven. Her daughter, Phoebe, now five, was only given a fifty-fifty chance to live. Her youngest, Joshua, was born with the umbilical cord around his neck. If he'd have been in any longer, he wouldn't have made it. Each pregnancy was tenuous and fraught with complications, including bleeding and traumatic preterm labor.

"It was just one thing after another!" Beth gave a lighthearted,

ain't-that-life chuckle, and swallowed. "I kept thinking, isn't taking
one enough? But I know that many people go through many more
losses, so I'm still blessed."

Through the near and actual losses, Beth came to appreciate that
a loss is a loss. Yet her understanding was not without contradiction.

"I simply cannot imagine losing my baby in my third trimester—
that level of loss!"

But she didn't let this feeling diminish the fact that the loss she
experienced was real.

As Beth intuited when she was younger, she and Jason were gifted
with kids with special needs. Jacob was unofficially diagnosed with
Asperger's syndrome, while Phoebe has muscle issues in her mouth
and couldn't communicate verbally until she was two years old. Beth
believes her miscarriage was meant to shape her as a mother. She
wouldn't be the same parent had she not lost Hope.

The children all know about their big sister. With Jacob now in the
first grade, several classmates' parents have asked Beth for clarifica-
tion about this confusing other child.

"Hope is in heaven, and she's a real part of our family," Beth
explains. "My son is proud that he has two sisters and a brother."

I wondered whether her children were ever asked those questions
directly. How would they explain the absence of an older sister who
never lived on this earth?

"When you're young, you just think that's how life is supposed to
be. From the moment they were born, we ingrained in them that they
had a sister. I've found that the older we get, the more parameters we
put on life and the more callous we become." Beth maintained an
upbeat lift to her voice with a smile to match it, but there was a fire in
her eyes. "I don't really care how uncomfortable it makes somebody
else. If I don't acknowledge Hope, then I'm denying her life. And even
though she wasn't here for very long, I need that."

Years ago, Beth was too emotional to have conversations with people who challenged her parenting or religious beliefs. But she said writing about the experience and giving her daughter a name helped solidify her convictions and gave her the strength to speak openly and proudly about them.

Beth was a bit shyer, however, about her affinity for psychics. Two separate clairvoyants made her question the understanding of Hope that both her aunt and grandmother's apparition had affirmed. The psychics suggested that Jacob, her oldest, was supposed to have come three months earlier, which was Hope's due date—and since that body wasn't viable, her soul had gone to the next child. Jacob, they explained, was really an embodiment of Hope.

While Beth didn't believe the psychics' musings to be the complete truth, she certainly relished her visits with them.

"I'm a weird Catholic," she said with a chortle, then scrunched up her shoulders and arched her brows, leaning in toward me. "They're fun, right?"

"Sure!" I was relieved to have this lighter, playful moment, an invitation to connect on a more personal level. I had a feeling Beth would understand my not-so-dirty secret of indulging in the occasional astrology reading. "It's a different perspective, like going to a therapist—everyone has their own lens."

"Exactly! And I wasn't sure about *their* particular lens . . . but they both said it!"

We both laughed.

"So if I get to heaven and it's different, who cares? The point is, for me and our family, it's real."

One morning, Beth sat down at her desk, put her hands on her computer keyboard, closed her eyes, and asked herself what she needed to capture on paper. What did she need to work through, and how could God help her do it? The writing, she found, helped her explore her faith and life experiences. She kept writing and refining, and after nearly six years she published a book.

"I looked back and realized that mishaps and misfortunes and challenges in my life—in everybody's life—are meant to shape us. I didn't realize that until I wrote this book," she said. "I just wrote for five years."

By the end of her writing journey, Beth had come up with a seven-step strategy to find perspective in life.

She could have used that perspective during the miscarriage to deal with people who didn't understand how to show up for her, she told me. Her in-laws avoided her and Jason. Her own parents didn't know how to communicate with her.

"I got upset because it felt like I was only good to them if I was producing a kid," she said.

When Jason called his mother out for her absence, she said she'd wanted to put a card in the mail but hadn't known what to write. People were so scared to say the wrong thing, they ended up not saying anything at all.

I asked what would have been soothing for Beth to hear, curious what role her faith might have played.

"Definitely not 'everything happens for a reason' or 'you'll get pregnant again.' Those are *my* truths! I *do* think it happened for a reason, and I *did* get pregnant again," she said. "But I just needed someone to say, 'I'm here. What can I do for you? Do you need a hug?'"

Beth discovered that if people weren't going to acknowledge her loss, she would have to do it herself. If that made people feel awkward, she said, shame on them.

As so many women discover, Beth found that sharing her miscarriage story invited others to talk about their experiences of pregnancy loss.

"Here in the South," she said, her voice growing louder, "people don't want to offend. But y'all need to get past that! This is real! This happened. I went through labor with no medication!"

I pointed out that it wasn't just her in the balance, it was also her family and her community. She wasn't the only one who needed people to acknowledge it.

"Even my husband!" she exclaimed, then looked down at her hands. "That's one thing I probably could have done better. When I think of the miscarriage, I think about what happens to the woman. But it was a joint experience." She said she wishes they had leaned on one another more. Jason was going through pain and grief too, yet not a single friend or family member showed up to support him.

That was eight years ago. Beth feels a lot has changed since then. There is still more to be done around normalizing the dialogue around loss and grief, she said—but in her world, at least, several changes have taken hold. By sharing feedback with her doctor and nurse practitioner, she played a key role in shaping policy at her Ob/Gyn's office. Now, instead of having women wait in the same room after their ultrasounds, nurses escort them back to the main waiting room with the rest of the patients. That minor change was a major step toward respecting patient privacy and vulnerability.

Beth's visits to that doctor's office since have largely been better, particularly when Beth was pregnant with Phoebe and dealing with intermittent fetal heartbeat. The medical team was doubtful she would make it to term. During one of those questionable ultrasounds, the tech hadn't said anything yet but Beth knew from the look on her face that the heartbeat was irregular. The woman grabbed Beth's hand and began rubbing her belly. "I will pray for you," the technician told her. "Good things to come, think positive thoughts."

"She knew!" Beth cried. "Just creating an environment where it wasn't over-promising but it wasn't all doom and gloom either."

Overly apologetic for having spoken for so long, Beth asked that I share my story of loss. I was reluctant to open up, afraid my sharing would impact what or how little Beth might share afterward—but then I remembered my vow to engage in honest dialogue around loss.

In retelling what happened and how I came to work on this book, I opened the door for the two of us to express mutual affirmation and empathy for embarking on our respective writing paths.

I had first connected with this chipper brunette in a business-women's group on Facebook. Beyond her home decor business and some cues about her Christian faith, I'd known little about Beth before meeting her today. I could not have imagined then that we'd have so much in common.

For most of her adult life, I learned, she'd worked in public relations and marketing for a major nonprofit organization. She kept feeling a stir within her to pursue something greater, she just didn't know what at the time. And then Hope came along.

Like me, she never planned to be an entrepreneur. She started doing home decor to help fund the book she didn't know she was writing until, half a decade later, it was published. Like me, she never intended to become a writer, or thought that her miscarriage would provide the inspiration and foundation for her writing.

For us both, writing about the experience has been cathartic, an avenue we've traveled across to get through the pain. We share a sense of responsibility to provide healing and support for others.

"When something happens to us," Beth reflected, "I feel we should submit to help somebody else."

Beth encouraged others who experience pregnancy loss to find an outlet. You cannot hold it in, she urged, whether that's painting or journaling or planting a tree.

"The moment you let it out, it's very freeing. It makes you realize that it doesn't define you," she said, chin upturned. "The essence of my book is that the only thing you can control in life is your reactions to it. So I try to look at life not as happening *to* me, but *for* me."

It took Beth a long time to adopt that mindset. She's been using it to find a way through her most recent challenge: the return of her endometriosis. Being pregnant and nursing all those years protected her against the debilitating symptoms for a time, but now they've resurged.

Her psychic told her it wouldn't be wise to have more children. Her doctor warned her that her body was no longer equipped—that she had pushed it to the hilt. She advised Beth to have a hysterectomy or go back on the pill.

Beth wasn't ready to deny herself the potential to be a mother again, so she opted for the medicine. She is on a continuous pill now, without periods, and she often doubts that this is the best course of action for her health. But she also knows she can't make the permanent decision yet to remove her uterus.

"I was actually more confident in who I was as a pregnant woman. That feeling of being strong and womanly. I remember having to overcome the pain, thinking that if I could grow a human, I could figure it out," Beth said, noting how she hadn't been able to overcome that pain as a teenager without the medicine. "So I've had to think long and hard about not having that option anymore."

After our conversation, I found myself lingering on the image of a strong, confident, womanly self. Did that have to come through pregnancy? Was fertility what shaped that image? Why do so many women let their strength and confidence be defined by successful birthing and mothering?

I thought about all this as Beth tried to make sense of her current situation. I felt the familiar ambivalence—or was it longing?—about having kids. Yet again, I saw myself reflected back to me in Beth's mirror.

"Maybe it's because I've lost that I can't put a permanent end to it," she considered.

Maybe that was also why I, nearing my fortieth birthday, still hadn't gone back on the pill. Did I fear it would throw off my body for too long to readjust to the possibility of pregnancy before my fertile window closed? Could I not shake the desire to experience the full range of womanhood? Why was I still clinging to this notion of idolized beauty and power in the pregnant body?

There were still so many maybes and what-ifs.

CHAPTER 12

Shirley

"Freeze your fucking eggs."

A WOMAN BEARING A STRIKING RESEMBLANCE to Victoria Beckham, with a gaze the intensity of Cher's, opened the door to her Oakland bungalow and greeted me with a warm embrace of slender arms and floral fragrance. She showed me into a small dining room, made even cozier by a sizable exercise bike opposite the table, where we sat down to talk about miscarriage and the virtues of freezing one's eggs.

"Listen," Shirley launched right in, boring through my forehead with her laser-focused eyes. "I consider myself to be a really open person, and I've been relatively open throughout the process, but when I've talked to friends about it, I feel like I need to have this exterior shell and pretend like everything's okay, when really this journey has been anything *but* okay."

It was my first hint of Shirley's spunk. After I assured her she was safe to drop the facade with me, she softened her eyes and relaxed her petite shoulders.

"I'm obsessed with pregnant bellies. I reach out and touch strangers whether they like it or not," she confessed, laughing. "I've been rubbing uteruses with pregnant friends, and I think it's magical, something I've always wanted to experience."

Shirley, thirty-eight, grew up in Israel and worked as an oncology nurse at a hospital in Marin. Nursing was her second career. She was in real-estate and mortgage business until the market tanked in 2007, at which point she lost everything: her house, her savings, credit, and her boyfriend. She had to start all over at thirty. Over the next five years, she was able to pull herself up, working full time and taking night classes. Right before her graduation, she traveled around the world alone for three months, learning how to enjoy her own company and live into her strength. When she returned, she met a handsome physician two years her senior, Niv, and immediately knew he was the one. They've been trying to have a baby since they got married three years ago.

Shirley knew many women trying to conceive, several of whom had done the full gamut of fertility treatments with varying success. Some of those struggling were much younger than Shirley, but she and Niv never worried for themselves.

"Maybe I was naive, thinking I wasn't going to have any problems," she said with a toss of her long, dark hair.

Shirley's parents, her "heaven and earth," were high school sweethearts; they married at eighteen and had her a year later. By thirty, they had three kids and were done making babies. They never went to college, and when they moved to the US to create better opportunities for their children, they immersed themselves in American culture. Here, they learned, young adults typically go to college, travel, and do all sorts of things before they settle down and have kids. So while Shirley described waiting to start a family until she was thirty-five as "sinful" in her grandmother's eyes, her parents were more understanding of the generational shift, particularly in progressive Oakland.

Shirley had been on birth control for much of her adult life. Once she was off, she and Niv spent a year trying without really trying. They had fun with it until it suddenly dawned on Shirley that she might not be able to make a baby on her own. It felt like she had failed this critical test of womanhood. She decided to make an appointment at the fertility clinic in her network.

"From the outset, I didn't really love my doctor. He was just checking boxes: I fit into *this* category, so now *this* was the plan," she said, looking like she'd just tasted something bitter.

Shirley found out that her uterine lining was thin and it was difficult for her body to create the follicles that mature into eggs released during ovulation. They decided to try intrauterine insemination (IUI), which was covered under her plan.

First, she was given all sorts of medications—oral and intravaginal, as well as trigger shots.

"I let my husband give me the first shot so he could feel like he was part of the process," Shirley said, snickering.

When she asked her doctor if they should keep trying in conjunction with IUI, the doctor said, "You can try as much as you want, but you'll never get pregnant naturally."

Shirley's jaw dropped as she relayed this to me. "It felt like I got hit by a truck! She made it sound so casual and nonchalant." Her eyes lit up and she wiggled in her chair. "But at least my husband and I could stop having sex on a schedule and resume intimacy for fun. It really took the pressure off."

When I asked Shirley if she felt Niv was part of the larger process, besides the obvious contribution of his sperm, she hesitated. "I think he was trying, but I still felt really alone. Even though he did and said all the right things."

Besides Niv, there were only a few people Shirley could talk to about her fertility issues: her best friend, who'd done IVF and recently had a baby; a work colleague she'd bonded with, who was also trying to conceive; and her mother.

She deeply wanted to discuss the issue with others but didn't want to be a burden. As an oncology nurse, who knew all too well the suffering of her patients, she felt she couldn't legitimately complain about her situation.

"This was just a little bump in the road," she said with a wave of her hand. "I didn't want to make it into a big thing . . . although it was really big to me."

Some women dread the self-injections the most; Shirley's biggest complaint, however, was the side effects from all the fertility meds: nausea, dizziness, fatigue, bloating, cramping, and weight gain.

I asked her if she was warned about those effects.

"Not really," she said, sighing. "I got a handout, but I did the majority of the research on my own."

Before starting the fertility treatments, Shirley was diagnosed with episodic depression and put on medication. Clinical depression and anxiety runs high in her family—"We're all medicated," she explained. She had just gotten over a hump with the depression when the fertility doctor advised her to come off the antidepressants.

Shirley refused. "I did not want to go back to how I was feeling before," she said firmly.

Her doctors ultimately respected her decision, and they forged ahead with the IUI. Once her follicles reached maturity, she was ready for the insemination. Niv was at work, so she drove there to collect his sperm in a sterile specimen cup.

There was a bit of confusion on Niv's part about orchestrating the sample, but Shirley was determined. "I don't care, babe, just get it in there!" she snapped at him.

He figured it out and Shirley, specimen in hand, raced back to the clinic.

"Everything lined up," she told me proudly. "Sperm count was great, cervix was wide open, follicles were big and juicy. The insemination part didn't even hurt. I sat there and read a magazine, put my feet up. When I came back home, I painted and used some creative energy to manifest what I was hoping for. And that," she said, wiping her palms, "was IUI round one."

Two weeks after insemination, Shirley was instructed to take a home pregnancy test. Staff had specifically advised her not to take it any earlier to avoid false positives. But she couldn't help herself.

She immediately called her best friend and shrieked, "Oh my God, I'm pregnant!"

"Shir," her friend said, "aren't you supposed to wait until Saturday?"

"I couldn't wait," Shirley explained. "I feel pregnant."

"That's great, honey, I'm happy for you," she said. "But you need to wait a few more days. I don't want you to get your hopes up."

Shirley didn't budge. She *felt* different; she knew she was pregnant. With bubbling excitement, she went to the drugstore and dropped hundreds of dollars on pregnancy tests. Each day, she took a test and saved them all inside a small Ziploc bag. It was the first time she'd ever seen the display indicate a positive, and she couldn't get enough of that rush.

"It was such a good moment!" She was radiant. "I started going on Pinterest and doing the whole baby thing. It was kinda crazy." She laughed.

When she told Niv just shy of the two-week window, he was cautious. From a physician's perspective, he expressed his doubts as diplomatically as possible to his ebullient wife.

Shirley, undeterred, called the fertility clinic a day early and told them she was convinced she was pregnant. A sympathetic nurse ordered the lab work and Shirley went in that afternoon.

"Having to wait twenty-four hours would have been agony," Shirley explained.

The nurse called the next day to wish her congratulations.

"I was sooo happy," Shirley cooed. "I was in my car, big grin on my face, couldn't wait to tell my mom."

She was so delighted, she didn't mind the nausea or exhaustion. She took the opportunity to enjoy a few weekend getaways before her pregnancy symptoms became worse.

Shirley and Niv had just returned from a trip to Santa Monica when she went in for her first ultrasound at eight and a half weeks.

"We were the talk of the clinic!" Shirley boasted from the edge of her seat. "Had people high-fiving us—first IUI, pregnant on the first try. Everybody knew us. We were walking on this beautiful, pink, fluffy cloud."

Shirley couldn't wait to feel her baby's heartbeat and hoped it would be a girl. Niv cautioned her not to get too excited as she changed into her gown and put her feet in the stirrups.

The midwife they had chosen came in and introduced herself, and instantly Shirley loved her. She was thrilled to know that this woman, whom she already felt so connected with, would be there throughout her journey and help deliver the baby.

The midwife started the ultrasound while Niv, a radiologist, watched intently.

As the minutes went by, Shirley's nerves kicked in.

"I looked at my husband, and he looked at me then looked down," Shirley recalled, the color draining from her face. "He never looks away. I just knew at that moment."

The midwife had a doctor come in to confirm there was no heartbeat. They told her they were sorry.

"I was disgusted with myself." Shirley practically spat the words out of her mouth. "I was so angry that my body couldn't create a happy environment for this beautiful bundle of cells that was supposed to thrive into a baby." Her sour expression intensified. "I imagined a black, rotting corpse in there."

She wanted it out immediately. But as much as she hated waiting, she decided she couldn't stomach a D&C—the risk of infection and scarring, having to lie awake while they scraped her insides. She wouldn't stand for letting it pass naturally either, though, since who knew how long that would take, so she opted to go home with the pills instead.

The midwife told Shirley to expect a few days of heavy bleeding and warned her the medication might not work, so Shirley got two sets of pills: misoprostol and mifepristone, both medicinal hormones that work by softening the cervix and triggering uterine contractions to prepare the body for labor. Shirley was to start the first set of pills that day; if she didn't start bleeding within five hours, she was supposed to wait a day and take another set of pills.

After calling in sick to work for the following day, Shirley lay down on the couch, downloaded a bunch of feel-good entertainment, and took the first pill along with an Ativan to ease her anxiety.

Shirley couldn't focus on the happy movies. She couldn't focus on anything. She sat on the couch, paralyzed by fear, wondering what she would see and feel.

Niv was working in his home office that day. He checked on Shirley periodically, reminding her each time that it took some women longer to respond to the medication. Hours went by, day turned into night, and the Ativan had made Shirley tired and groggy. Lying in bed, she figured the pill was a dud and planned to take the back-up medication the next morning.

"I didn't think about wearing a pad or laying down a towel because I assumed it wasn't working."

Shirley paused and I laughed nervously, unsure of how her emotional pendulum might swing.

"Well, it worked!"

Shirley woke in the middle of the night in a pool of blood. She had bled through the mattress. She didn't wake Niv. She went to the bathroom and sat on the floor.

"It was fucking awful," she said, barely a whisper. "I remember thinking, *Oh God! This is what women go through all alone, in their bathrooms. This is what it's like to lose a baby.*"

Shirley discussed the matter as if it were years removed; she didn't shed a single tear. Yet her pain was palpable in the way she leaned in, clutched the table, and drove her words into me with her taut lips and unrelenting eyes.

"I was so deeply in my loss. I had attached myself to this idea and just like that it was gone," she said, leaning back in her seat.

In a hushed voice, she told me it took her over a month to miscarry completely—and I let out an "Oh my gosh!" without even realizing it. I was transported back to white-knuckle nights of shooting pains and groan-worthy cramps that consumed me for nearly three weeks. I couldn't imagine having gone through another week of it.

"Every day it was a fucking reminder of my loss," she said, her hands balled into fists. I was right there with her. "Every day. And the clinic had completely dropped me. There was no need to follow up with me."

I echoed the notion I'd heard from so many women: "You become a non-patient."

"Exactly. You're not pregnant, you're a loser! Moving on to the next person who's successfully pregnant!" She threw her hands in the air. "No follow-through."

Shirley had recently visited so many medical professionals—fertility clinicians, the midwife, her regular Ob/Gyn, and her primary doctor—and now she wasn't sure which of them to turn to. She figured someone would want to do an ultrasound to confirm the fetal tissue had passed. Yet nobody bothered to check in.

She read some blogs that made her feel less freakish about the protracted bleeding. Then one day, she woke up with terrible vertigo from all the blood loss.

"It was as if somebody took the world and shook it," she told me. "I lost all control."

She'd developed vestibular migraines associated with postpartum hormonal shifts. She didn't feel comfortable driving and called in sick several times.

After suffering with headaches for weeks, then the sudden dizziness, she finally went to her general practitioner. The doctor did a CT scan and full physical, but the only advice she gave her was to increase her iron and fluids until the bleeding subsided.

Niv booked a trip to Hawaii a few weeks into the miscarriage as a salve for Shirley's pain. The morning of their flight, Shirley was in the shower, soaping up, when she reached between her legs and felt something strange come out of her. When she looked down, she saw the fetus in its full form. This was five weeks after she had started miscarrying.

Shirley called for Niv—"Get in here!"—and held up the bloody mass for him with shaking hands.

"What the hell, babe?" he said. "Throw it away!"

"This is it, right? This is it!"

Niv jerked her hand over the toilet and flushed away the fetus. "Don't do that to yourself."

The experience gave Shirley closure to a certain extent; it was finally out of her and she could move on. But she didn't know how. She sank into a deep depression. When people asked how she was holding up, she'd act like everything was fine. "Like I didn't just go through some fucking marathon!" she joked with me.

She felt sad and isolated. She shut herself off from the people closest to her; she stopped working out. She would come home from work, pour herself a glass of wine, and zone out in front of the TV. Too steeped in her grief for intimacy, she even disengaged from Niv.

I asked her if she felt any hope or interest in trying again.

"Not at the time," she said flatly. "I was thinking more, like, *Fuck, I'm gonna have to do this again?*"

Shirley toggled between self-loathing despair and buck-up affirmations, reminding herself that infertility and loss were just part of being a woman. "People do eleven rounds of IVF, this is just one miscarriage," she would say to herself. "Come on, get your shit together."

She tried seeing therapists, but she didn't feel like she could open up, not even with one who'd also suffered the loss of a child. But she knew she had to turn things around for herself.

With a smile, she pointed to the exercise bike in the corner and announced that was the moment she had bought a Peloton.

The bike was a catalyst. Shirley was eating healthier and staying active, physically and socially. She felt back in her body and in control of her life. Eventually, she felt ready to try a second round of IUI.

Shirley shifted awkwardly in her chair and asked me in a higher-pitched voice if I wanted to hear more. I was rapt.

"I'm pregnant right now," she said, nearly giggling, then looked out the window. "But my baby's not growing. Again. I just found out a couple days ago and . . ." She looked back at me with blank eyes. "I feel nothing."

Entirely taken aback, I told her how sorry I was to hear that. Shirley had first contacted me about sharing her story a month earlier but ended up canceling our meeting when something came up. She must have circled back as soon as she found out. I couldn't believe she'd invited me over in her current state.

"It's okay," she replied, waving her hand.

"It's not okay," I said, smiling.

"It's not okay," she agreed.

We laughed.

Shirley was six weeks along, and her HCG and progesterone had plateaued. The fertility clinicians were still monitoring her, worried about an ectopic pregnancy. She would have to go in for another ultrasound and labs, though not for pregnancy purposes—rather, to figure out the safest way to miscarry.

I asked Shirley, in her numbed purgatory, how the medical community might improve care for women like her. What would be a

better experience, given the lack of follow-up care with her first miscarriage and what she was going through now?

"I just feel like there should be more," she said, letting out a huge
sigh. "More communication, more education, more support."

She suggested that practitioners pair patients up with women
who recently miscarried so that they could discuss their experiences
together. She had discovered some local support groups for grieving
mothers outside the medical field, and she said the community sharing had helped to normalize her pain and suffering, and allowed her
to connect with others.

Shirley hadn't told anyone about the recent news besides Niv, her
mom, and now me. This time around, they'd decided against telling
people she was pregnant. With the last pregnancy, Shirley had given
Niv's mother, who was eighty and craving grandchildren, a quirky
gift to announce that her dream would come true—one of the many
positive test sticks from that Ziploc baggie. When his mother realized
what she was staring at, after a comical near-encounter with the tip
where Shirley had urinated, she burst into tears and threw herself on
the couple, showering them with congratulations. Now they regretted
giving her that false hope, and had vowed not to repeat their mistake.

Shirley's family in Israel was encouraging her to move back to
take advantage of the free IVF she would receive there as a citizen.

"Sure, but what do I do, leave my job? How badly do I want a baby?
Badly enough to put my career on hold?" Shirley shook her head.
"IVF feels irresponsible of me."

Shirley hasn't let go of the traditional notion of adulting: get married, buy a house, have a baby. Since recovering from the crash and
marrying Niv, she's been working on building a big enough cushion
to buy a house in the Bay Area, where the median house price has
more than doubled in the last five years.[11]

"I don't know if I'm holding back or just enjoying what's available
to me. Or maybe I've just gotten to this place where it's not all dreamy

and perfect; there are some real struggles." Shirley relaxed her gaze
and almost smiled. "I'm tired of swimming against the stream. I just
want to put my hands up and go with it, see where it takes me."

Knowing how fresh the news was, I wanted to know what advice
Shirley had for other women dealing with pregnancy loss. Would she
be able to take her own advice? I had the familiar feeling of leading
a coaching session, gently guiding a client toward her own solutions.

"Freeze your eggs in your twenties," she said. "My girlfriend just
turned thirty, and asked me what she should do for her birthday. I
told her, 'Freeze your fucking eggs. Do you want to have children?
Freeze your eggs.' Why not? Why wait?"

Shirley wishes she'd frozen hers.

"I don't want to tell her she might have difficulty, but you know
what? That's life! I have friends in their late twenties, early thirties
having trouble getting pregnant. It's not just an age thing, there's a
variety of reasons. But any woman who knows she wants to have children? Freeze your eggs!"

As our conversation grew to a close, I had the sense Shirley didn't
want me to leave. She nearly convinced me to get a Peloton after
walking me through some of her favorite cycling instructors. She
also said she was worried she'd slip into another funk and have to
watch the bike collect dust.

When she asked if I wanted to see the studio where she painted,
I obliged, curious about this aspect of her life she described as so
joyous and fulfilling. As we entered the light-filled room off the
garden, I felt her heaviness melt. Her paintings were full of color and
life—curvaceous women lounging in the sun, vibrant flowers bloom-
ing from the canvas.

CHAPTER 13

Katie

"Life seems so much more fragile now."

DAN WAS SET TO PROPOSE on top of Mount Kilimanjaro. The plan was simple. He had the ring sewn into the harness of his paraglider that he and Katie carried up in multiple pieces. The moment they launched, he was going to ask.

As they neared the summit, the cold wind strengthened; as they set up along the edge, the weather turned brutal. Instead of making the leap, a blizzard set in and they ended up camped out at 19,000 feet for three days.

Once the storm let up, Dan popped the question.

"Even the most beautiful and best-laid plans don't always work," Katie told me.

We sat at a bookstore coffeehouse near Katie's home, northeast of San Francisco. She was thirty-four, married for five years, and had recently suffered a major loss. I studied the attractive, olive-skinned brunette. She smiled with her big hazel eyes and a soft curl of her lips, her long hair and wispy bangs framing a classic Grecian face with a becoming mole on her right cheek. She looked like an off-duty Pilates instructor, equal parts granola hippie and sporty chic.

Katie and Dan are still avid adventurers. When they met ten years ago, they weren't interested in having children. They felt a childfree future better suited their active lifestyle.

On their first anniversary, they sailed their boat to Cabo, Mexico. They used to spend every Christmas there together on their little sailboat, until, after a few years of marriage, Dan announced that he was done with that holiday tradition. "I'm really bored with our life," he told her. "I want this to be our last Christmas without a family."

Katie, looking out at the ocean, the horizon open in all directions, agreed. She signed up for one child. Dan had two brothers and his mother was the sort of über-maternal figure who adored children and vigorously celebrated the growing ranks of her grandchildren. Dan pushed for three, but Katie was firm. "One kid," she said. "We'll see where that takes us."

The following Christmas, Katie was eight months pregnant with her daughter Sophie.

The pregnancy was wrought with complications. For the first six months, Katie had such severe hyperemesis—an extreme form of morning sickness—that she was unable to keep fluids down and had to be hooked up to an IV. Even without solid foods, there were days when she threw up thirty to forty times. It was altitude sickness and seasickness wrapped in one. After the second trimester, the sickness finally subsided and she was able to gain weight. The rest of her term was normal until six weeks before her due date, when she went into prodromal labor, with pseudo contractions every ten to fifteen minutes.

As we spoke, her eyes softened. "It was horrible. I couldn't function."

I asked her how she managed the pain.

"How does anyone? I was so set on having a natural childbirth that I wouldn't let them do anything."

Katie hired a doula, who turned out to be a huge disappointment. When Katie called asking what to do and wondering if her experience was normal, the doula would tell her, "This is *your* normal," or "Well, it's happening to you. If it's happening to you, then that means that it happens." Katie found neither comfort nor guidance in these responses.

Hoping for more, she hired a midwife, but it was a group through her medical insurance, so she met with a different person every visit. The midwives didn't communicate with one another about her condition and the care was inconsistent.

At the time, Katie was running her own business, working in finance for renewable energy projects. She was in the middle of a big financial closing, pulling long hours. One day, in the middle of a call with an investment banker, she began to feel contractions. She excused herself as the pain rose inside her; when it reached its summit, she jumped right back on the call.

When she finally went into active labor, Katie was five centimeters dilated and contracting every minute for sixty hours. Dan, her parents, and the doula were all at the hospital, but at some point the doula sent her parents home because she thought Katie would be staying much longer.

"So my parents left," she said, giggling, "and the doula fell asleep." The doula had sent Dan out of the room to sleep too.

Suddenly, the heart-rate monitor flatlined. Katie read the monitoring nurse's grim expression: the baby's heart had stopped. Doctors quickly prepared her for an emergency C-section. Within five minutes, baby Sophie was out of Katie's body and her heart rate had stabilized.

"The night before I had the emergency C-section, I was laboring without drugs for the third day with nobody there." As Katie spoke to me, her voice dropped to a whisper. These moments, anonymous and safe as we were in a busy coffee shop, are still those in which we feel we must hide our shame.

As soon as doctors got Sophie breathing, they put her on Katie's chest to breastfeed, with Katie still cut open. They discovered the birth had been so complicated because Sophie had been tangled up in the umbilical cord and unable to descend. The cord had been wrapped twice around her neck and three times around her body. In an effort to comfort Katie, the doctors assured her, "Well, the good news is this will never happen again. This kind of thing never happens twice."

Sophie was a difficult infant, but they eventually settled into their rhythm with her. As Dan began to express his desire for more children, Katie had more and more doubts about growing the family. Finally, they agreed not to talk about a sibling until Sophie was two years old.

Then, after visiting friends who had a three-week-old, Katie told Dan she didn't think she could do it again. She couldn't imagine having to contend with the sleep deprivation or countless challenges she'd faced with Sophie.

Dan was crestfallen. He yearned for another baby, but he respected their agreement. They would stick with one.

After a picturesque family hike on Father's Day that year, Katie felt ill and started throwing up. "For a week straight, I puked my brains out. Like, *What did I eat?!*" she recalled, laughing. "Just thinking it was food poisoning. My mom was like, 'Katie, you're pregnant.'"

Katie was in denial. She genuinely wondered if she might be allergic to cheese. Her mother insisted she was pregnant; to prove her wrong, Katie decided to take a pregnancy test. She tested positive and soon found out she was already eight weeks along. Sophie was only fourteen months old.

Her lighthearted mood shifted before me as Katie told me how upset the news of the pregnancy had made her. "I cried," she nearly whispered. "I called my husband thinking he would be upset too. I even told him, 'Sit down, I have some horrible news'—but he thought it was the best!"

Once Katie heard the excitement in Dan's voice, she succumbed.

As soon as she let herself get swept up in the expectant buzz, the hyperemesis struck again, only this time it was even more extreme. She was sick for nearly four months, hooked to an IV, completely laid up. The genetic testing and twenty-week ultrasound came back normal, and eventually the sickness subsided and she was able to gain weight. Throughout the pregnancy, Sophie breastfed and slept poorly, adding to Katie's exhaustion.

As if the pregnancy weren't stressful enough, Katie was in the process of selling her business and setting up a consulting firm during the first trimester. She had just signed contracts with a host of new clients, but realized early on that she wouldn't be able to manage the workload. She was too sick. She dropped all but two of her clients. Looking back on it, she realized how crucial that decision was for her. "I ended up doing exactly the work I wanted instead of worrying about who would pay the best or what would fill my time," she said.

Meanwhile, Sophie learned sign language for "baby" and was growing increasingly excited to meet her younger sibling. "Seeing my daughter with my belly was so sweet, hugging and feeding it," Katie recalled with sparkling eyes.

Two days before Thanksgiving, Katie was practicing yoga with Sophie, doing a downward-facing dog, when she felt the baby completely roll over in her womb. She hadn't experienced such dramatic movement before and couldn't shake the feeling that the baby was stuck in an odd position.

That night, she dreamt she was running from the Grim Reaper with a tiny baby in her arms.

Dan woke her up when she started screaming in her sleep; Katie stayed awake the rest of the night, sensing something was off. She had felt the baby roll over, but no subsequent movement. When she got up in the morning and still hadn't felt any activity, she and Dan decided to go to the hospital to get things checked out.

She was twenty-six weeks along.

At the hospital, a nurse did a doppler ultrasound and didn't hear anything.

"As soon as she was searching around my belly for the heartbeat, I knew what had happened and started sobbing. I was inconsolable because I had just become so excited about the pregnancy," Katie said, choking up. "Our kids would've been exactly two years apart . . . In your mind, you build your whole life around what this child is going to bring to your future . . ."

While the nurse went off to find the doctor, Dan told her, "It's going to be fine, their machine's just broken."

The nurse returned with the doctor, who did another ultrasound and confirmed there was no heartbeat. The cord was completely restricted, obstructing blood flow to the baby.

It was a nightmarish reenactment of Sophie's birth two years earlier—only this time, the baby didn't make it.

"They didn't even check my record the second time," Katie managed between sobs. "Doctors really ought to have sensitivity training."

I remarked how painful the doctor's false reassurances from years earlier must have felt as I rummaged through my purse for tissues—to no avail. In my rush to get out the door, it seemed, I had forgotten them. I felt awful.

As I stood up to find some napkins, Katie shooed me back down.

"Between my cold . . ." She paused to sniffle and pulled a small cloth from her bag.

"And your small child," I said, smiling.

"And everything!" She laughed and blew a strand of chestnut hair off her damp cheeks. "I never go anywhere without wipes."

The hospital staff told Katie to go home and do whatever she needed to do to say good-bye. She could come back whenever she was ready to be induced to deliver her stillborn child.

I asked Katie what that was like.

"I thought, how could they let me out of here? How can they tell

me to go walk around with my dead child inside me? How can . . . ?"
She looked off in the distance, patting her eyes, then turned back to
me. "I was so angry."

She remained furious until she got home and began preparing for
delivery. She changed her clothes and packed a labor bag for the hospital. She took a picture of herself in the mirror, her big belly bursting
from the profile. In hindsight, she said, she was grateful to have had
that moment.

Dan stayed with Katie throughout the hospital visits. Sophie was
with her nanny until Katie's mother arrived from Colorado that same
day. Sophie had never gone to sleep without her mother before, so
Katie tucked her in and waited until she fell asleep before they left for
the hospital to be induced.

The doctor had told them it would take twelve hours to deliver.
Katie thought they'd just be there overnight—that they would be
home before Sophie woke up.

She was in labor for thirty hours.

"It was awful," she whispered, shaking her head. "Just knowing
you're in labor and your baby's dead, and you still have to go through
it all."

Dan was a wreck during labor, muttering to himself and pacing
the room. Katie, meanwhile, was focused on the task at hand, doing
whatever she needed to get her stillborn baby out of her body.

"I really kept it together," she said in her matter-of-fact, stoic
manner. "Then, after it was all over, we had to plan what to do with
the body. That's when I fell apart, and my husband took over and
was the strong one." She took a deep breath and exhaled. "Because I
couldn't deal with that."

Katie delivered a girl weighing two pounds. The nurses swaddled
her and let Katie hold her, then put her in a little bassinet next to the
bed. Katie and Dan hadn't known the sex until she came out.

"I just wanted two little girls so bad. So bad," she said, her body contracting with each quiet sob. "I remember looking at her and imagining her getting big. I couldn't accept that she was gone."

Katie sat there with her for twenty-four hours, convinced her baby would come back to life.

"It was bad; it got to the point where her skin was peeling off, and I still couldn't accept it," she said, looking down.

The hospital was used to parents like Katie and Dan. Unlike with miscarriage, there was an established protocol for stillbirths. The staff set them up in a room in the back corner of the ward, its door marked with a small leaf so others would know to give them privacy to grieve. The nurses also gave them couple a small keepsake box, took the baby's footprints, and gave them the little hat they'd put on her to take home. They let them keep the blanket she was wrapped up in and even helped with the funeral arrangements. Katie felt they did as much as they could.

One nurse, however, seemed to have missed the memo about the stillbirth. When Dan walked out into the hallway, she greeted him, "Congratulations, daddy!"

Dan shot back, "Don't come near my wife."

They had the body cremated. Katie found an artist online who turned some of the ashes into jewelry: two necklaces, one for herself and one for her mother.

Dan went right back to work. Maybe it was just his way of coping. Katie took much longer to get back to working, mothering, and living. Physically and emotionally, she went through the usual postpartum changes, only this time without the newborn. When her milk came in, her daughter Sophie, who was still breastfeeding, didn't quite know what to do with it all. Katie decided to donate it to someone in need.

"I thought it would feel good to donate. And then, when the woman was coming to pick it up, I just couldn't get out of bed," she said softly. "It felt like I was giving away the last piece of her."

Dan ended up meeting with the woman's husband to hand off the milk. Although Katie never actually met her, she heard that the woman had been pregnant at the time and had delivered a healthy baby. She had a medical condition that prevented her from producing her own milk, so she was thankful to have Katie's.

"I feel good about it now," Katie said. "The physical aspect was really hard. It's still hard! With my first daughter, even after the C-section, I really didn't have any trouble getting back to my activities and losing weight. With this past pregnancy, I haven't gotten back to my normal self yet."

Three months after losing the baby, Katie returned to work on a part-time basis so she could spend more time with Sophie.

"Life seems so much more fragile now." Katie stopped bothering to wipe away the tiny rivulets flowing from her eyes down to her chin. "I'm really grateful."

I struggled to grasp Katie's gratitude. Was she willing herself to be grateful as a sort of coping mechanism? I wondered how I would feel in her shoes—my life upended, facing such traumatic loss. Could I be that strong?

"I'm grateful for the perspective," Katie said. She also said she was grateful for the time with her daughter. For her health. For where she is now in life.

"More than anything, I've learned the depth of my emotions and the depth of love that I'm capable of. Just treating life as a miracle. I was never one of those people who would say, 'Oh, a baby is a miracle!' It's biology—animals do it, we all do it. It can't be a miracle; otherwise, we would not be here." She paused, her face aglow. "But now it really is!"

The experience of loss changed Katie's outlook on life. Now she desperately wants to have two children, the irony of which is not lost on her. But she isn't quite ready to try conceiving again, she said, knowing full well that the next pregnancy, with its inevitable hyperemesis, will be intense. Plus, given her high risk of cord accident, they'll have to do invasive cord monitoring.

"I've put this one in nature's hands." A perfectly arched eyebrow lifted as she shrugged. "We're not *not* trying, but we're not tracking my cycles and that kind of thing, so we'll see."

Katie said her biggest challenge in coping with the stillbirth has been the isolation.

On a recent family outing to a museum teeming with expectant mothers, Katie's spirits sank. When she shared her sadness with Dan, he told her she ought to be grateful for what she had.

"Being sad doesn't mean I'm not grateful for my daughter!" she told me, leaning forward in her chair. "It's not one or the other."

Overall, though, Katie feels the experience brought her and Dan closer together, especially during and immediately after the stillbirth. They learned to lean on each other more than they ever used to. Because of all the outdoor activities they shared together, they had a very physical, obvious way that they would rely on one another, but not so much a spiritual or emotional reliance. Through the loss, they were able to build that aspect of their relationship.

Yet the tension around grieving remains a challenge.

"When he tells me to be grateful, I don't just sit down and listen. I tell him, 'Please don't say that to me. That is not an appropriate thing to say to somebody who's grieving,'" Katie said, with an air of calm about her. "And he listens."

On other occasions, however, Dan has been less empathetic—at Christmas, for instance, with Katie's family. It was just a month after the loss.

"You don't need to talk about what happened," Dan told her. "Don't make this all about you."

"Excuse me?" Katie said to him, horrified. "What am I supposed to do, just pretend nothing happened?"

"Just go on like it's a regular holiday," he tried.

"It's not!" she gasped.

Dan was worried she might turn the festivities into a funeral.

Katie acknowledged that her husband can't always give her his full support, nor should he have to. Fortunately, there are a handful of close friends and mothers of friends who have held space for Katie in her grieving, particularly those who've had similar experiences. She's grateful to those women for making themselves available to sit with her and letting her know it's okay to feel sad.

"Day to day, it's hard to go through the emotions alone. Sometimes when I'm sad, Dan will tell me he still thinks of her—that he's sad, too. But he's had a much easier time getting back to normal."

Katie struggles with the discrepancy between Dan's healing and her own. She half-jokingly suggested that the real trauma for Dan was losing his adventure buddy, though she was far from smiling when she made the remark. Katie had to quit paragliding and other strenuous activities they used to love as a couple for a while, though they're starting to get back to it now.

"It seems we have even more fun now doing it with our daughter, bringing her along on our little adventures," she said with the sing-songy tone of a teacher at story time.

But she also said that Dan's tendency to pack their days with hiking and biking all over town—getting back to their usual couples activity status—could be overwhelming for her. Her body hadn't completely recovered, and the waves of emotions often left her feeling outpaced.

"The experience has been a dramatic slowing down of my entire lifestyle," she explained. "I don't necessarily want to go back to rushing from one activity to the next. I'm ready to sit still for a while."

The woman Katie hired as a new doula for her second birth sat with Katie afterward and confided that she too had suffered a traumatic pregnancy loss. The doula reminded Katie that even when she felt alone, she wasn't. Healing, she said, was non-linear.

"It's okay to feel like your old self one day and then the next to feel totally miserable that you lost your child. There doesn't have to be a rhyme or reason to feel the things you're feeling," she urged Katie. "You just have to feel them."

For Katie, this idea—that there's no schedule for healing, for the return to normalcy; that some days will be better than others; that it simply takes as long as it takes—was both soothing and affirming.

In an effort to feel less alone in her grief, Katie signed up for one of the nationally acclaimed Return to Zero retreats, tailored exclusively for women who have experienced the loss of a child. Katie looked forward to the meditation, group therapy, and deep-healing opportunity the retreat in the mountains would provide her. There would be yoga, too, but she was a bit apprehensive about that part.

"I used to do a lot of yoga, and I think because that's what I was doing when everything happened, I haven't been able to do it since. I don't know if I'm mad at yoga," she told me, lightly blushing. "It's been such an integral part of who I am for a very long time. I'll get back to it eventually."

Katie didn't express regret, per se, with doing yoga during her pregnancy. Her only real regret—and source of guilt—was not being more excited about the pregnancy from the outset.

"In my heart," she started, her puffy eyes welling up again, "I know that this isn't true, but there was a while where I wondered if the child heard me say that I didn't want the pregnancy and chose not to be here based on that. But I know that's not reality."

Katie felt that we would all stand to gain from talking more about pregnancy loss, especially those suffering alone and battling feelings of guilt. I asked her why she thought it wasn't something we talked about socially, and why society buries the subject in whispers.

"Because of the patriarchy!" A smile exploded on her face. "Because of misogyny! That's why we don't talk about this."

It seemed pat, and yet I couldn't disagree. I wondered, could it be that simple?

"We need to elevate all women's issues. We don't allow women to make decisions about their own bodies, and then we don't allow them to talk about it!" she exclaimed, her eyes growing wider. "Taking away their rights, then even their ability to talk about their rights!"

I suggested that if this were a men's issue, we'd be hearing about it.

"If this was something that men struggled with," Katie said, with a clever grin, "then there would be open-mic night talking about pregnancy loss! Every comedian would talk about it."

To be fair, I've seen men grieve pregnancy loss too. Dan himself admitted as much, though it looked different. While the existing support for women is far from adequate, there's dramatically less such support for men. Katie's upcoming retreat, for instance, was only for women facing loss, not for parents or fathers. Boys learn at an early age that they should avoid expressing their emotions, which complicates men's ability to discuss and receive support for grief.[12] Perhaps because of that, relatively few men might attend a retreat or support group to discuss their feelings about pregnancy loss. If men's bodies were implicated in pregnancy loss, Katie suggested, then we'd be having a much more open conversation about these issues. Women's bodies and experiences of trauma remain taboo, however—shrouded in shame, mystery, and silence.

Women deserve more credit for being able to talk about loss, as painful as it may be. "Understand that we're stronger than that," Katie said. "We can talk about it and not be a mental case."

Katie became far more vocal as she healed. When people asked her if Sophie was her only child, Katie replied that she was her only living child. At the same time, she was careful not to idolize or elevate her deceased child.

"I bring it into my day-to-day dialogue," she said. "It hurts every time I say it, but it hurts a little bit less the more I normalize it."

Dan had a hard time accepting Katie's openness to discussing the loss. For him, it was too much—too hard, too painful. He preferred not to talk about such matters.

"He really wants to talk about the good things, and that's fine," she said half-heartedly.

"That's fine when things are great," I offered.

"Yeah, but it's not real," she said, shaking her head. "It's the most human experience you could have. But we only want to talk about these fake things that we've constructed. We don't want to talk about what makes us real humans."

After we hugged good-bye, I watched in a half-trance as Katie set off in the other direction, her muscular body moving gracefully through space. I admired the vulnerability she'd shown in speaking her truth. In the late afternoon sun, her silhouette appeared strong and solid, and recalled the strength and resilience I've seen in so many women moving through their grief and beyond.

CHAPTER 14

Miranda

"I can't believe it's still like this!"

When Miranda first got pregnant, she wasn't thrilled.

"*Oh my God, I don't want to have a kid!*" she recalled thinking, shrieking. "*What the heck am I doing?*"

Miranda was thirty-four and had been married to Jeff for six years. "I was just on the cusp of being an ancient person in terms of having a baby," she deadpanned. "In the medical world, I was legitimately dead already."

We hadn't spoken in over twenty years, but Miranda was still the fireball of sarcastic hilarity that I remembered from high school. We were in a grrrl band together then, and Miranda played drums like Animal from The Muppets.

Miranda and Jeff lived in a modest home in New Jersey, near where we grew up on the Shore, and taught dance at a local studio. I imagined her zaniness and infectious laugh afforded her favorite-teacher status amongst her students.

After her Ob/Gyn confirmed she was seven weeks along, Miranda joked, "I'm not really pregnant though, right?"

"Oh, you're definitely pregnant," her doctor said.

While she and Jeff weren't trying to conceive, they weren't being particularly careful about things either. Miranda wasn't all that surprised when she found out, though it wasn't until she heard the heartbeat that her disbelief dissolved. With that tangible connection in place, her enthusiasm for having a baby bloomed.

Miranda shared the news with about a dozen friends and relatives. "I didn't know you weren't supposed to tell people." Her pitch rose, taking on the tone of an awkward question. "I thought just as soon as you get pregnant, you're supposed to say, 'I'm pregnant, yay!' Nobody told me about miscarriage."

Like millions of women, Miranda was not aware of the unspoken twelve-week "rule" about not announcing a pregnancy until the second trimester. Given higher rates of miscarriage in the first trimester, many wait to tell family and friends—although a growing number of advocates for women's health question this standard, as secrecy around early pregnancy means that women who miscarry tend to grieve in hushed isolation, stripped of support from health-care providers and their own social networks.[13]

Miranda went back to the Ob/Gyn for a routine check-up a few weeks after her initial appointment. She lay on the exam table as the technician did the ultrasound.

"It was the one where you have to drink a bunch of water so that your bladder pushes against your uterus, so when they check you it's closer to where the embryo is," she told me, straight-faced. "And you're about to pee all over everybody, which is so much fun."

The technician kept circling back over Miranda's belly, checking a second and third time. As the room grew quieter, Miranda had a bad feeling. Eventually, he told her he couldn't find the heartbeat.

"Well, try harder because I'm really excited," she told him, half-laughing, half-sighing. "Couldn't find it? Cool, I'll wait. Go on, probe me."

Miranda's smile waned. The technician kept saying, "I'm so sorry," as she clutched the crinkly paper beneath her, hoping he wouldn't give up.

Afterward, she lay alone in the exam room for what seemed like an eternity before someone told her she could get dressed.

"I was hysterical, crying, when they finally brought me into my doctor's office. While I sat there waiting for her, I heard her talking with someone in another room about their burgeoning pregnancy," she said. "It completely messed with me."

When the doctor came in, she told Miranda she was sorry and there was nothing that could've been done to prevent the miscarriage.

"It is not your fault. This is very common," she assured her. "It's so common that it's probably happened to you before and you didn't even realize it."

"Okay, but . . ." Miranda hadn't passed any of the fetal tissue. "It's still inside me, right?"

"Yes," the doctor said. "Here's how we can go forward: you can get a D&C, which is where we take it out, or you can wait for it to pass naturally."

"This sucks so bad!"

Her doctor nodded. "I know, it totally sucks."

Miranda opted to wait and let nature run its course.

"Honestly," she told me, "I don't really like procedures, so I just wanted to let it pass." She paused, and her big green eyes grew even wider. "But that's a lot easier said than done."

When Miranda left her doctor's office that afternoon, she hadn't fully accepted the loss. As the week wore on, she felt a nagging urge for someone to double-check for the heartbeat. She felt too embarrassed to go back to her Ob/Gyn, so she visited a local Planned Parenthood office. The staff there confirmed that the fetus was dead and presented her with the same options: get a D&C or wait it out.

As soon as she left the clinic, she called her doctor to schedule the procedure.

"It was so hard knowing that the thing wasn't living inside me," she said, looking away. "I just couldn't do it."

She had the D&C a week later.

For Miranda, it wasn't an issue of trusting her doctor. Her Ob/Gyn was no-nonsense but compassionate. Miranda wanted to believe her, but she wasn't ready to let go of the baby she had grown so excited to meet. She wasn't ready to accept the loss. And like so many others, she felt guilty about the miscarriage. "I was convinced I shouldn't have danced . . . or whatever I was telling myself."

Miranda's doctor told her she could try again after having a regular menstrual cycle, but that time came and went. She wasn't in the headspace to jump back in. She spent the summer trying to reconnect with herself.

"I remember walking to a friend's house—just me, alone—and wanting to feel powerful and good about it, not all sad because I was panicking."

She wanted to know for herself that she could be okay alone, without a child to care for or a baby growing inside her. She wasn't a big drinker, but it felt important to know she could go have a drink if she wanted. She needed to feel positive about herself, on her own, before bringing yet another soul into her body and psyche. She took her time.

Come September, Miranda felt comfortable enough in her own skin to start trying again. By late October, she was pregnant.

I asked if they shared the news this time around.

"Oh, hell no!" she cried. "Because that next time I knew how to do it."

Miranda was about six weeks pregnant when she tested positive with her home kit. Two days later, she started cramping and bleeding. Despite the positive test result, she wasn't sure if she had just gotten her period or was actually experiencing a miscarriage.

Her doctor didn't mince words. "There's no such thing as 'kind of' pregnant, Miranda. You were pregnant."

Miranda miscarried again, but she said the experience was far less crushing the second time around. Aware of how common it was, she didn't feel nearly as bad about the loss. She reminded herself that she'd have more opportunities to try again.

"It wasn't the end of the world to me like it was before. I knew that if it ends itself, it's really not meant to be," she said in a practiced tone. "If you think about it scientifically and pragmatically, it's not as torturous. You know, nature taking care of itself."

Miranda was able to pass it naturally, but she was unprepared for the extreme amount of pain and blood loss. She bled heavily for a couple days, then her flow became more like a period for the following week.

"It was unpleasant, to say the least," she recalled, shuddering. "But I was grateful that it happened early, and I was more prepared for it mentally." She threw her hands in the air, palms up, and shrugged. "I mean, it's crazy! The human body's insane!"

We lamented our personal and societal lack of understanding of women's reproductive anatomy, reminiscing over some embarrassing formative instances of ignorance.

Miranda, recalling the first time she got pregnant, burst into laughter. "I had to read up on it! ō-vyu-lā-tion." She patted her eyes. "I'm thirty-five, I've had my period for twenty-four years, and I'm like, 'So the egg comes out of where?' It's so lame!"

When I asked how Jeff coped with the losses, Miranda's whole body sank.

"It was difficult for him, and it actually makes me sadder to think about his experience than mine. He's so quiet that thinking about him suffering makes me feel worse."

Tears gushed down her pale cheeks.

"He was awesome . . . and very quietly there for me." She sniffled, shaking her head. "I remember him asking me what I'd want to watch on TV—something that would last a while. And he just went and bought all of *Parks and Recreation* for me."

They watched a lot of *Parks and Rec* together, allowing themselves the comforts of comedy and easy entertainment.

When Miranda asked Jeff how he was handling the loss, he would tell her how sad he was and remind her that she wasn't alone. "We understood each other, and I didn't feel abandoned emotionally or physically. He was really there for me," she said, her eyes welling up again. "He's a really good dude. I found a good one."

A couple months after the second miscarriage, Miranda and Jeff were ready to try again. They got pregnant right away with Maggie.

"The third time really was a charm," Miranda said, grinning widely.

A cherubic little brunette popped onto my screen and whispered, "Hello," squirming in her mother's lap to avoid eye contact with me. I could see Miranda's high cheekbones and pointed chin in Maggie, as well as her playfulness.

Seeing Miranda in full mom mode, I asked how she'd felt about womanhood and motherhood around the time of the miscarriages.

"This idea of 'fertile' womanhood is cut off at such an early age," Miranda said. She understands there are real biological factors at work but said society also plays a significant role, insinuating that women themselves are no longer viable after a certain age. Thirty-five years old was considered late in life for Miranda to be starting to conceive, but that's how long it took for her to feel like she was ready to care for another person.

I noted that many women feel like they've been written off when they hit their mid to late thirties.

"Right!" Miranda cried. "The message is, 'You waited too long. Why did you care about other stuff more than this?'" She contorted her face into a mock grossed-out look, then relaxed into a dream-like expression. "I've never felt so womanly as I did when I was trying to get pregnant, or was actually pregnant. It made me feel more in touch with my femininity, in a way, whatever that means anymore."

She chuckled. "Those parts are there for a reason! They're there, they work, and they have this crazy, intricate function that I had not even considered until then."

Miranda said that even during the traumatic experiences of loss, she saw the inner workings of her womanly body as beautiful and wondrous. "It's amazing that my body knew that it wasn't gonna work and made the call to let it go. It really teaches you about loss just by virtue of it working."

Miranda said she wished the people to whom she announced her first pregnancy had warned her against sharing the news so early—but in the same breath, she acknowledged how hard it is to discuss the possibility of loss with excited friends and family. "I've had friends since then tell me they're six weeks pregnant, and I say, 'Yay, that's great!' But all I can think is, *Why did you tell everyone so early?!* I know what might happen! On the other hand, I wish there was more info and intel about miscarriage." She gasped and threw her hands up in the air, looking around wildly. "Seriously! I can't *believe* it's still like this!"

The contradictions Miranda felt point to how and why the conversation around early pregnancy loss needs to shift. If women felt supported when they experienced pregnancy loss in the first trimester, maybe they wouldn't shy away from letting people know about their early pregnancies in the first place. Because there's so little support or understanding of the impact of early loss—heard in comments like, "She wasn't even showing"—the standard of twelve weeks makes it that much harder for women to speak up and find support.

"You should be able to tell people that you're pregnant and then, later, that it didn't work out," Miranda argued. "Even before you can hear a heartbeat."

I asked Miranda why she thought, as women, we're not talking about it.

While she couldn't put her finger on it, she did feel that miscarriage should be more than a mere footnote in the book on pregnancy.

When I pressed her about what would have actually resonated with her, she lit up.

"The information should be there as soon as you find out you're pregnant." Her hands whirred at her sides. "It should come with pregnancy tests! Once the thing turns positive or you hear, 'Congratulations, you're pregnant.'"

She was having a stroke of public health brilliance.

"Remember that miscarriage is a really high probability." I listened intently as she tried to pace herself. "You know those TSS [toxic shock syndrome] warnings in tampon boxes that basically said, 'Don't leave this in for a thousand years, or else'?"

I nodded, vividly recalling how effective those warnings were. As a teenager, I was terrified of TSS, which occurs in about one in every 100,000 women who wear tampons.[14] To put that in perspective, miscarriage is about 25,000 times more common than TSS.

"It should be in every pregnancy test kit! There should be a pamphlet that gets sent out anytime you might be pregnant: 'It may not work out. And if it doesn't, it wasn't your fault. It wasn't that drink you had when you didn't even know you were pregnant. It's not that your body sucks, or you're not female enough, or you're too old to do this. It happened because your body's taking care of you.'" She paused, then added, "Anything! Just more information, preventively."

She had similar thoughts about what might have helped Jeff feel more supported.

"There's advertising on the Internet for just about anything you'd ever want to buy. So why can't there be something targeting men, like, 'Hey, are you guys trying to conceive? Are you a dad-to-be? Here's what you need to know.'" She started giggling. "But make it look cool so dudes actually read it."

Miranda acknowledged that not every male partner is as

empathetic or as kind as Jeff. She was adamant that men should understand that supporting their partners through pregnancy also means supporting them through a loss.

"In fact, your support is monumental if it doesn't work out. I can picture, slash I know, what happens if your partner is less sensitive and you lose multiple babies. It's not easy to deal with shaming, in addition to feeling the loss. So, I think sensitivity training would be important, too."

Miranda was full of public health and education suggestions for policymakers. I asked her what advice she had for women who have struggled with pregnancy loss as she has.

She leaned back in her chair and let out a big sigh. "No matter how crappy things feel, even those crappy experiences can be a lesson." Eventually, she said, we remember even the low points in a positive way, as impossible as it may seem at the time of our suffering. That memory and lived knowledge, she believed, enables us to help others and find solace for ourselves.

"Even if you never have kids, you'll experience motherhood in other ways," she said, her heart-shaped lips broadening into a smile. "From the second I conceived, to birth, till Maggie and I find each other in another realm—the whole thing of being a mom is so incredible. Watching her grow is the coolest thing in the world. I appreciate it so much it hurts," she said, simultaneously laughing and crying. "I love the babies I've lost, and I love her."

Miranda's tight little frame heaved to the rhythm of her sobbing. She apologized as she caught her breath, "I was doing so great, I'm sorry."

"Please don't apologize for expressing such love," I replied, feeling my eyes water up. Miranda's bewilderment about her love of motherhood had ever so slightly loosened my grip on finding peace with not having children.

"Yeah, it's heavy," she said. "I just appreciate talking to you about it so much."

I thanked her for sharing so openly with me.

"It should happen more. It should just be a normal thing . . . but maybe your project will start it!"

I'm still beaming at the thought of this.

CHAPTER 15

Deven

"We're transformers."

Deven's first pregnancy loss was the single most empowering experience of her life—a complete validation of her intuition and self-knowledge.

She was at around nine weeks gestation and out of town for a work trip when the cramping and bleeding started. She'd known something was off the night before when she'd felt an unfamiliar pain in her back; now she went to the nearest ER, where the staff was clinical in confirming, but not confronting, what they saw in the ultrasound. Finally, they looped in her midwife, who affirmed Deven's suspicions: she was miscarrying.

It wasn't until this moment that Deven cultivated an appreciation for her mind-body connection operating on a deeper, more instinctual level. As the pain electrified her uterus, she was able to find comfort in knowing her intuition had guided her toward the likelihood of loss.

She moved through the pain, breathing into it with every jarring contraction—her yoga teacher training serving her in ways she couldn't possibly have imagined when she began her studies years earlier. Passing the fetal tissue was so viscerally acute, it seemed every nerve in her body was firing. Her earlier instincts helped her find acceptance and transcend the intensity of her physical being.

Miscarriage was common—Deven knew this already. She and her husband, Dan, had heard at least a dozen stories from their own mothers, other relatives, and friends who'd been open about their losses. They both understood it was just something that happens.

"I knew we were in the sea of life," Deven explained over Zoom, shrugging her broad shoulders. "It didn't make it easy, but it didn't make the uncomfortable feelings any harder."

It was refreshing for me to hear how cognizant Deven was of pregnancy loss prior to her own experience. It had caught the vast majority of others I'd spoken with by complete surprise. Deven's awareness had spared her the more common negative feelings of guilt, shame, and isolation.

Searching online for resources, Deven was underwhelmed. The religious perspectives so readily available on the web felt inaccurate and unhelpful. The belief that life begins at conception did not resonate with her.

"There's a lot about 'Jesus held my hand and face,' and such," she shared, rolling her eyes. "But I don't actually know there was ever a baby. I know we got pregnant, that it was really amazing to be pregnant for a couple of months, and then we were *not* pregnant."

Deven, thirty-nine, had known she wanted kids since her early twenties. But when she first met Dan, seven years her junior, he wasn't interested in kids. The second year they were together, he told her someday, maybe, he might be interested. The third year, it was a solid maybe, but he didn't think it would be with her.

"He actually tried to break up with me." Deven groaned. She looked like she'd just stumbled out of bed, wearing a mostly buttoned flannel, her hair a messy pile of blond locks, dark frames accentuating the rings under her eyes.

She told Dan she was in love with him—that she was a better

person because of their relationship, that he had to stay, that they were in it together. Dan knew she was right. They've been married now for five years.

Six months after Deven's miscarriage, she was pregnant again. This time around, the couple went through the wringer with Deven's hormonal fluctuations.

"I want chicken," Deven announced one afternoon—one hand crossed to her opposite elbow, the other covering her chin in a subtle betrayal of her confidence of this request.

She wasn't showing yet, but the symptoms were blaring. Dan was doing his best to support her, encouraging her to stay active and not mope around. He knew her history of clinical depression. He was cooking for her, too, or at least attempting to. Deven was increasingly picky about her cravings, and Dan was indulging her particular brand of crazy as much as possible.

One day, he suggested a dish he knew she loved.

Deven gasped. "God, don't do that!"

"What if I roast it with potatoes and mix up a salad? That's always good." He was trying.

"No!" Deven looked at him as though he'd just suggested eating dog food. "Definitely not that!"

"Okay, so maybe I'll just boil the chicken."

For the next three days, she ate boiled chicken. On the fourth day, when he put a plate of it in front of her, Deven wrinkled her nose.

"Dan, this is gross. Why would you make that for me?"

Soon, she was throwing up daily and the fatigue was weighing on her. She could barely function. As a yoga instructor, she was aggravated by her inability to maintain a regular activity level or any semblance of a mindful presence.

Her mind, in fact, churned over whether the intensity of what she was experiencing meant it was a viable pregnancy. She figured it must. She certainly wanted it to be.

At around eight weeks, Deven and Dan met with a few midwives and settled on a nurse practitioner they felt was a good fit. The following week, Deven would have her first ultrasound.

A week before the appointment, however, Deven had an especially rough day. Once she finally motivated herself to get off the couch and go for a walk, she felt a rush of fluid leave her body. She was in a frenzy when Dan got home later, worried about the blood loss in an otherwise healthy pregnancy. When she phoned her Ob/Gyn, the doctor explained that it's not uncommon to bleed during pregnancy.

Since she didn't seem all that concerned, Deven tried to let it go—but couldn't. Her mind drifted into analysis. She didn't have any of the cramping she'd had with the first miscarriage, so she ruled that out. In fact, her body hadn't offered any of the clues she noticed before. She did the "Doctor Google" thing, and the symptoms checked out as a few conditions she didn't recognize or the possibility of twins. With the daily vomiting, unusually rapid weight gain, and highly specific food cravings, she was convinced it was a baby, if not two.

The next week, on the ultrasound screen, Deven and Dan saw an undefined blob. No little gummy bear, no heartbeat—just a mass.

The nurse reassured them that they hadn't done anything wrong, then referred them for a more intensive ultrasound.

The lab tech, accustomed to excited couples awaiting this advanced imaging, greeted them cheerily. They had to explain that it wasn't that kind of situation.

Deven was relieved she had asked Dan to go with her. Her shock was tempered by his usual calm and groundedness.

The staff collected all sorts of lab work, but nobody would explain what all the fuss was about. Occasionally, someone would mutter about this or that result not lining up, then announce a new test to run. Eventually, the medical staff sent Deven and Dan home without any further insight as to what to do or expect, saying only that her doctor would follow up with them as soon as possible.

In the meantime, Deven and Dan distracted themselves by watching movies, reading light fiction, and curling up together by the fire.

The doctor called the following week, over Christmas break, dispelling Deven's theory of twins. It was a molar pregnancy, she told her.

Molars are similar to ectopic pregnancies, in that the condition indicates that something went wrong along the way. There are different kinds of molars; in Deven's case, the sperm had fertilized an egg without any DNA. Similar to the experience of having twins, women with molar pregnancies commonly experience unexpected bleeding and grow much more quickly.

As much as it felt like a pregnancy, there had never been a baby, let alone twins. It was all there in Deven's womb, everything in the right place, but the cells that create the placenta had gone unchecked.

"Your readers absolutely need to know this," Deven said, sizing me up. "Are you ready?"

I leaned in.

"Sometimes there is no baby!" She paused, then repeated the words. Then she explained that wanting others to understand how crucial this issue is for women's health is what motivated her to share her story.

Now that they understood it was a molar, Deven's doctor explained that they would need to remove it, immediately. It was so urgent, her doctor had already booked a D&C and cleared her schedule for that very afternoon so she could meet Deven at the hospital. This was the same doctor who, days before, had told Deven to make an appointment for two months out "just in case."

Since the couple was in San Diego with Dan's family for the holidays, Deven went to a nearby hospital. Her Ob/Gyn made all the arrangements with the medical team there.

The night before the procedure, Deven and Dan treated themselves to an early sushi dinner. The morning of, they rose shortly after dawn to leave for the hospital.

"We might need to do a blood transfusion," said a man in scrubs as they prepped Deven. "We'll just need your verbal consent."

"Sure, if you need to do one," she said.

"Actually, we might need to do two," he said, hooking up another tube. "Given the vascular nature of the uterus and the size of the mass, we're not sure how difficult it will be to remove. We might need to stop the blood flow to the uterus, and if that doesn't work, we'll have to take it out."

"Take what out?" she asked.

"Your uterus."

Deven looked over at Dan and said, "Hon, we're really good at the little stuff, and I think we're about to get a lot better, because who knows what's going to happen when I wake up from this!" Then she turned back to the doctor. "So, basically, everything will be okay as long as I don't bleed too much, right?"

"Yeah, that'd be great!" he said, then put her under.

The procedure took under an hour. The mass they removed was the size of a softball. Deven had measured fourteen weeks when she was only nine weeks pregnant.

Deven spent the next two weeks recovering in the bosom of her extended family. They fed and pampered her, not even allowing her to get up for water. Though she wouldn't be having a baby—sometimes there is no baby!—at least she had solid support and a fully intact uterus.

Back home in Bend, Oregon, she went in for a routine checkup and broke down wailing in her doctor's office. Dan was with her as she was diagnosed with postpartum depression. The therapist on call told her she wanted to meet with her weekly to make sure the depression didn't become clinical. While Deven was already taking a lot of the right steps, the therapist encouraged even less screen time, regular rest, a healthy diet, and as much yoga and meditation as possible. She explained that before the D&C Deven's HCG levels had been off the charts, similar to what occurs pregnancies with twins, and after the D&C they'd bottomed out—along with her spirits.

Deven immersed herself in teaching, which provided a refuge from the dark stories she was spinning in her head. She was grateful to have the studio and the opportunity it offered her to shift her attention and energy toward others who looked to her for guidance and support. Her depression lifted, and the lab testing was scaled back from weekly to monthly.

Dan had just left the country for a long-awaited adventure in Patagonia when, on Valentine's Day, the doctor left Deven a message saying she'd made an appointment for her first thing Monday morning. That's when she got the diagnosis of gestational trophoblastic disease (GTD).

GTD occurs when abnormal cells grow inside the uterus after conception, and it can develop into malignant brain, lung, or uterine cancer within months. Of the 0.1 percent of all pregnancies described as molar, roughly 10 percent evolve into the precancerous GTD.[15] Deven's older age—thirty-five when she got pregnant—may have elevated her risk for developing these rare conditions.

Instead of making a baby, they had effectively made precancer.

Doctors instructed Deven to start chemotherapy right away and told her she'd likely be in treatment for six weeks. It ended up being eight. They warned that the chemo might make her angry, but she was mainly exhausted. Determined to overcome the adverse effects, she was careful to avoid stress and get enough rest.

She was on her way to the gynecological oncologist in Eugene, a few hours' drive from her home, when her Ob/Gyn phoned with the news: Deven's HCG had hit zero; her body at last understood it wasn't pregnant. The cancer specialist confirmed that her levels looked good and helped her piece together the medical events of the last half year. She was finally in the clear.

Finding the couple's new normal, post-chemo, was bumpy. It took a while for Deven's appetite to return, which threw off her energy over the course of the day. The treatment was especially hard on her liver, and the rage and aggression she'd been warned about during the treatment but never experienced suddenly surfaced in that following month.

One afternoon, she barked at Dan, "I'm really angry right now!"

"Okay." Dan's voice was steady and familiar.

"I just want you to fight with me!"

Dan smiled. "Babe, I'm going to make you a sandwich."

I noted how amazing her husband sounded.

"Yeah," she said, blushing, "Dan's pretty great."

A year later, when they got the green light to conceive again, Deven was all in. She had been waiting for this moment, anxious to get back on the baby-making track.

But Dan, between sobs, told her he didn't think he could do it, at least not yet. As she held him, letting his tears dampen her hair, she gently pushed for an explanation.

"I didn't know my options were: baby, no baby, dead wife," he told her.

It's common to withhold our own emotions when we're helping others through crisis. Once they move out of crisis mode and don't require as much support, then caregivers can have their moment. This was Dan's. It was only now that Deven was healthy again that he could finally begin his own processing.

He suggested they enjoy the summer, without the pressure to conceive. Deven didn't press the matter. She knew they would have to figure out what they needed, as partners. The trials they'd gone through with the chemo and pregnancy losses had helped them find their path. Now they would have to be patient and make sacrifices for one another—the essence of partnership, in Deven's eyes.

Dan, for instance, had said he would never get a dog. Ever. Period. But when he was in South America and Deven was in chemo, she started fostering a dog. About a month in, the dog went up for adoption, and Deven wasn't quite ready to part with it.

"Hey, honey?" she asked in her sweetest voice.

"Get the dog," Dan told her, shaking his head. "God. You're in chemo."

Autumn came and soon enough they were pregnant again. Deven tried not to worry about whether it would be viable.

"I never fantasized about what happens next," she told me. "A lot of people do, but I don't recommend it."

Deven didn't buy any baby stuff during the first or second pregnancy. With the third one, she knew how different it felt, but she mostly tempered her excitement. She didn't share that sense of unbridled joy she'd seen some of her pregnant friends espouse.

"That's just not in my wheelhouse," she explained.

Deven and Dan were careful about the language they used—"We got pregnant," they said, or "There's a fetus." They never called the first or second pregnancy a baby.

While she was cautious about not becoming attached to any one outcome, Deven really wanted a baby. She knew she wasn't up for IUI or IVF. If the pregnancy didn't work out, they would likely look into adoption.

When she was just ten weeks along, she splurged on some baby clothes at a local children's boutique. She couldn't help herself.

Universe, I'm really ready for this, she thought, walking through the pastel-colored aisles. *This is the one! I'm getting shoes and some onesies right now that are super cute. Please let this be a baby!*

Throughout the pregnancy, she was diligent about self-care and tried to channel her inner peace. For her, that meant meditation, bubble baths, and guided yoga nidra to fall asleep. She listened to her body and slept when she was tired. She knew Dan would cook for her, and this time she was better at articulating her needs. They applied the lessons from past pregnancies and moved through it more smoothly.

Fortunately, the Universe heard Deven's call—as evidenced by little Geo, who now appeared next to his mother on my Zoom screen. Deven was in extreme sleep-deprivation mode when we spoke. Three nights earlier, seven-month-old Geo had decided he would no longer sleep unless he was touching one of his parents. His teething only added to the exhaustion. What's more, those darn cute teeth had earned him a reputation for biting adults.

Deven was already nostalgic for that newborn time, which she described as a magical fourth trimester. Her yoga business was thriving by then, so she'd been able to afford to take a full three months off work. She'd listened to her gut and ignored the advice not to have their family visit, and ultimately felt she couldn't have chosen a better way to recover and acclimate Geo to their world.

Deven ended up having a C-section. She was a forceps baby herself, and other women in her family had gone the surgical route as well. She lamented the procedure and how much fear, in general, exists around birth. For her, she said, it was more about harnessing that power.

"We're transformers," she said, her chest rising. "The womb has the capacity to make life or death. It's a gateway."

Deven had stood at that gateway; she knew her power to transform.

If more of us were in touch with this power, I wondered, would we still suffer alone in the face of loss? How might we collectively harness that transformative power to uplift one another, and ourselves, out from the depths of our pain and loneliness?

CHAPTER 16

Rose

"Bottom line is, we were killing him."

Rose hit her stride around the thirtieth hour of labor. She lay with one hand over her enormous belly, the other over her heart. Bleached bangs plastered her sweaty forehead; hazel eyes closed to the blue glow of hospital equipment in the dimmed room. Deep breathing, like fairy dust, sent her into fleeting spells of slumber. She was over the hump now, beyond the first waves of exhaustion. *Breathe, sleep, breathe, sleep.* She focused her breath on her baby boy's last peaceful moments in her womb.

When she got pregnant at nineteen, Rose felt the dark clouds of grief begin to lift. Heroin had recently taken her older brother's life. A baby promised distraction, joy, and purpose. It might even reign in her mercurial boyfriend, Matt, nine years her senior, who ran in similar substance-fueled circles as her brother. Rose didn't know what to expect, but her body guided her every step of the way: No more cigarettes or junk food or suicidal thoughts. It was time to grow up and start acting like a mother. As she became more in tune with her body, she opted for a natural delivery.

At the thirty-sixth hour, the midwife's patience wore out. She was envious of Rose's naps and decided it was time to move things along. She broke Rose's water—and immediately, the baby went into shock.

A doctor squeezed Rose's hand, jolting her from her meditative state, and announced an emergency C-section.

Nurses barked at the midwife, "What the hell were you thinking? She's going to die!" while Matt lobbed her with expletives.

Once Rose had delivered Orson, she didn't want to let him go. Joyous relief mixed with a lingering fear of losing him—but her body needed rest. Each time she looked to Matt to hold the baby, however, he was slouched in a pink pleather chair in the corner, snoozing.

"You would've thought *he* was the one who gave birth!" Rose said, chuckling. "I threw tissue boxes at him, begging him to wake up." The nurses tried to stir him, but the best he could manage was a confused look and a mumble before dozing off again.

"The support was never there—for anything." Rose sighed. "We were gonna split up before Orson was born."

Though the delivery went well, Rose ended up with an infected incision, a blackened hole the size of a nickel. The nurses warned her, "Don't be surprised if you never feel anything down there again."

My eyebrows froze in steep arcs of shock. "Really?" I gasped. "That's rather life-changing news to hear."

"Yes!" Rose cried. "But the incision healed fine."

When Rose relayed the nurses' comments to the surgeon who'd performed the C-section, he assured her that she would retain the sensation in her sexual organs. She appreciated his confidence and sought him as her OB for her second pregnancy, at age twenty-two.

At her nine-week ultrasound, the doctor told Rose the fetus looked a few weeks behind. He prescribed a week of progesterone to boost growth, but Rose could only stomach the hormone for three days— it was debilitatingly exhausting. Her OB pressed her to get another ultrasound to check fetal development.

Rose was devastated to learn there hadn't been any growth.

"I felt so emotionally invested," Rose told me, looking down at her hands. "I'd already pulled up pictures of baby outfits and picked out names . . ."

The OB recommended that Rose get a D&C to clear out her system and avoid risk of infection. Knowing his patient preferred the natural route, he offered the alternative of wait and see, but advised waiting no longer than a week before acting.

I asked Rose how she dealt with the heartbreak when she left the OB's office. Did she have any support?

She smiled, thinking of her father, who had passed away just months before our call. "Dad was disappointed because he knew about my relationship. Like, 'You're already struggling, why get pregnant now?'"

When Rose explained that the pregnancy wasn't viable, her father offered his condolences and wished her the best. Yet the undertone was clear: why have another kid with *that* loser?

Rose saw past Matt's inability to show up for her. Losing a child, however, was not something she could easily absorb. Her mind swirled, parsing out what she'd done wrong.

"Did the doctor ever say it wasn't your fault?" I asked.

"Yeah, he was the only one, and it meant the world to me."

Still, Rose went home racked with guilt. "Completely self-hating," she described, the roots of which traced back to being abused as a young girl.

She came to see the miscarriage as a sign.

"It was nuts, but I really believed it meant we needed another kid together." Rose, now thirty-seven, threw back her head, laughing at her younger self. "I was twenty-three, in a tumultuous relationship since I was sixteen, and he's a decade older—so delusional!"

"I suppose you were pumped up on pregnancy hormones and emotionally scattered," I offered with a shrug, smiling.

"Oh my gosh," Rose droned, her irises disappearing in an eye roll,

"I was crazed! All that mattered was having a baby. I felt my partner wasn't there for me because I wasn't enough."

I had met Matt over a decade earlier, when Rose and I both lived in Oakland. I'd glimpsed then how terrible things were, as their relationship neared the end—and I'd seen Rose's dedication as a mother. She carried herself with a quiet confidence in a ballerina's lissome body, decorated with colorful tattoos and an understated nose piercing.

"Well, you're a wiser woman now—"

"Thank goodness!" she exclaimed, then drew her features taut. "It's taken much longer to understand that the abuse is now the past. I have a choice not to react like a six-year-old. I have a choice to make conscious decisions. But at the time, I thought, *If we get pregnant, then I'll be loved.*"

Rose was grateful to have Matt's company at the D&C. "That's the trick," she said, shaking her head, her caramel locks swishing across her chest. "They always give you just enough to keep you hanging on."

Four months later, Rose was pregnant with their second son, Faunus. This time, the pregnancy symptoms were especially intense, including strong aversions to bread, cheese, and meat. Rose was a celiac—but undiagnosed as such at the time. Before her pregnancy with Faunus, she'd regularly eaten gluten and endured sharp stomach pains after most meals. During this pregnancy, she stopped eating wheat entirely and felt great. She took it as further affirmation of wanting another child with Matt.

Rose's surgeon advised her to schedule a C-section. In fact, he told her if she wanted a natural birth, she'd have to see a different doctor.

"I wanted a natural birth, but I was scared," Rose told me. After Orson's birth, her mother had shared that she and Rose's aunts, grandmother, and great-aunts had all had issues with dilation. Rose figured it would be safer to have the scheduled surgery, though she bemoaned the harshness of the medical so-called convenience. "Nowadays, with so many C-sections, we have this idea that they're no big deal," she explained, "but it's actually major surgery and recovery."

Once Rose saw Faunus wiggling on the ultrasound, she was able to shake the fear of losing another pregnancy. "The kid wouldn't stop moving. It was obvious he would be okay," she said with a satisfied grin.

The C-section went well—a cheerful affair in the operating room, with music and laughter. Baby Faunus had entered the world.

Now Rose had two boys to tend—without a father's support. Matt would leave for work, saying he'd be back that evening; then he'd be gone days or a week. Sometimes he would say a week but be gone for two months.

Before Faunus's first birthday, Rose decided she'd had enough.

"That's it," she told Matt. "We're done. I can't continue on like this. I'm moving."

Matt picked at some dirt in his fingernail. "Okay." He looked up from his hands and flashing her his most charming smile. "Wanna watch TV?"

"No!"

Rose packed up the car, grabbed her sons, and left for Albuquerque.

In Albuquerque, Rose met Patrick, who quickly proved a dedicated partner and loving father to Orson and Faunus.

Soon after marrying, the couple had their own child together, Gabriel, via natural delivery. They were eager to keep growing the family.

"Honestly, I'd just keep having babies," Rose said, laughing. "I love kids!"

She was pregnant again four months after delivering Gabriel. She tested positive three times at home, but her OB's result came back negative. Rose requested an ultrasound, but the nurse insisted she wait. The next week, Rose was ravaged when she got her period. "I wanted to be pregnant and believed I was," she said.

Within months, she was pregnant—and hopeful—again. "A fresh reminder of how quickly things can change," she told me.

After testing positive at her OB's office, Rose asked for an ultrasound. Sensitive to Rose's recent loss, the doctor agreed. She returned shortly with a behemoth from the 1980s, its plug the size of Rose's head. After fiddling with the settings for ten minutes, her OB apologized, "It was the only machine I could wheel in, sorry. I have to move on to other patients, but we'll get you in next month, okay?"

As deflated as she was, Rose understood. The 2008 recession had hit Albuquerque hard; the clinic's outdated equipment was a reflection of the city's economy. She would have to wait for her twelve-week visit and focus her energy on a happy, healthy pregnancy.

Focus was hard, though, with three boys and a recurring nightmare that threatened to burst her aura of calm. In the dream, she would arrive at the five-month ultrasound and hear some version of "It's gone," or "The baby's massively deformed. You can't have any more children." Nightly, she woke in a sweaty panic.

To counteract the bad dreams, she practiced positive affirmations. Holding her belly, she'd whisper, "Everything's okay, we'll be fine." She reminded herself that pregnancy fears were normal.

Rose had always had remarkable dreams and premonitions. "In the rare dreams about people I know, they always express to me that something's wrong. When I wake up and check in with them, I find out something bad actually happened—the dream was right." She paused and drew a sharp breath. "It *sounds* crazy, but it's true."

As a teenager, Rose had glided into homeroom on the first day of high school in a new district and begun introducing herself—"Hey, so you're Jim," "You must be Laurel," "Alicia, right?" When her classmates responded, "What the heck? How did you know my name?" Rose told them she'd dreamt about meeting them a couple of nights before.

Given all this, she couldn't shake these inauspicious pregnancy dreams; she trusted her slumbering visions. She was torn between competing desires to acknowledge it wasn't "just a dream" and to adopt a more optimistic outlook. Rattled as Patrick was, he comforted her, "I know you're anxious, but let's try to be positive. For the baby."

For the twelve-week visit, Rose went to the state-of-the-art teaching hospital at UNM. She lay at a half-recline, her thighs spread wide, her feet in stirrups, excited to see the wondrous being in her womb. She drew her knees together when three men in scrubs shuffled into the small examining room. Each muttered greeting was more awkward than the last.

"These gentlemen are learning the ropes today." The middle-aged obstetric nurse smiled warmly at Rose, a touch of desperation in her voice. "Do you mind if they assist with the ultrasound?"

"Suuure, go ahead." Rose smiled politely.

The residents, eager to cut their teeth, took turns moving the wand over her belly but couldn't obtain any decent images. The nurse encouraged them to try transvaginally. *Geez, really?* Rose thought, opening her legs. *How hard can this be?*

The nurse guided the men while Rose focused on her breath, hoping to quiet the embarrassing questions and shuffling of feet.

After twenty minutes, the nurse grabbed the wand. "I'll take it from here." The room sighed with relief. "Looks like you're not as far along as we thought," she said, pointing out the undeveloped landmarks.

Rose's heart fluttered at the blurred glimpses of the creature's beauty.

"We'll just adjust your due date back two weeks," the nurse told her.

Rose left the hospital with renewed optimism. Yet the nightmares persisted. During subsequent prenatal visits at her clinic, she pleaded for an ultrasound. Each time, either the machine malfunctioned or none was available. Nurses assured her, "Listen to that strong heart! Your baby's fine. Next checkup, we'll do the ultrasound."

The highly anticipated five-month visit was scheduled at the teaching hospital. Finally, Rose would get to see her baby again.

After a lengthy search for parking, she and Patrick entered a waiting room swarmed with swollen bellies, children kicking in their seats, and anxious fathers-to-be. A flustered receptionist pointed the couple down the hall to an exam room.

"I'm so sorry we're late . . ." Rose began as a nurse rushed through the door.

"Lie down on the table, lift your shirt, and pull down your pants," the woman snapped.

Rose and Patrick exchanged glances as Rose undressed.

The nurse furrowed her brow and focused on the grayscale moonscape on the screen, moving the wand across Rose's belly like one might rifle through a purse looking for Chapstick—roughly, quickly, sighing in audible frustration. Then the wand froze and the nurse's lips parted.

Rose cleared her throat. "Is everything okay?" She felt Patrick's fingers entwine with hers.

"I have some questions. I'll get the doctor." The nurse slammed the door on her way out.

Patrick squeezed Rose's hands. "Everything's okay," he said softly.

Separately, they wondered, *How bad is it?*

Rose closed her eyes, simmering with animosity toward the nurse. *How rude! Like I'm some sort of deli sandwich to assemble, not a human being concerned about her baby's health . . .*

She tried to find compassion.

The doctor greeted the couple with a sympathetic smile and pulled down a large projection screen.

"Rose, you've seen your share of ultrasounds as a mother," she said, as the blown-up image appeared.

Rose nodded, holding her breath.

"Here you see the head." Pointing to a fuzzy blob, she explained that the skull hadn't formed around the brain. "There's no abdominal wall, either, which is why, here, we see the guts floating. There the spine is twisted."

Tears fell down Rose's cheeks as she absorbed the information. With so many anomalies, there was no way the baby could survive. Its heart still pumped, but who knew for how long.

"So, you know this isn't what we typically see," the doctor concluded.

"Yeah," Rose whispered.

"Please. Let's get you cleaned up and talk in another room."

A nurse showed Rose and Patrick into a conference room down the hall with a table, four chairs, and a box of tissues. While they waited, the baby's beating heart echoed in Rose's head—sounds of life and feeling. She shuddered with the thought that keeping him in her body might cause him pain.

Rose's doctor joined them to discuss the bleak options: deliver a stillborn baby or undergo a dilation and evacuation (D&E). Rose floated above the conference table, moving in and out of the recurring dream that had so haunted her—and proved prescient.

The doctor explained that carrying the baby to term would likely require a C-section; as a rule, doctors don't perform more than three in a woman's lifetime. Rose had already had two C-sections, so future conception would be medically inadvisable.

Rose wasn't prepared to give up having another child with Patrick. She was only in her early thirties, with plenty of time to expand the family. More pressing was the matter of harm.

"We felt more comfortable with the D&E knowing his pain would end . . . *if* he was feeling it." Rose paused, her lips slightly parted. "Bottom line is, we were killing him, but it was compassionate."

The word "kill" landed heavily for me. Rose hadn't been acting out some cruel intentions; she'd been heartbroken, weighing her unborn child's suffering.

"He was alive, this living being," Rose explained. "I wasn't afraid of the procedure; it was the fear of harming him versus hoping he'd somehow be okay."

Once Rose accepted that things wouldn't improve with the pregnancy, she felt a mounting urgency to stop her baby's potential pain. She scheduled the D&E for the following day with Chella, one of the "angel doctors" who'd helped deliver Gabriel.

Chella described the procedure as a simple outpatient surgery that wouldn't take more than an hour and a half.

Because of the dreams, Rose hadn't announced the pregnancy. Even her sons hadn't noticed it, despite her obvious growth, so the only people who knew were Patrick and her mother, who happened to be visiting.

While Patrick looked for parking the morning of the D&E, a thought flashed through Rose's mind: *You're going to die.* She quickly reassured herself that she'd be picking up the kids from school in a few hours, and the worst was already behind them.

Rose warned the anesthesiologist that her body processed anesthesia quickly, relating her excruciating experience after bearing Gabriel, when she felt the doctor massage her uterus under the false assumption that she was still fully under.

"Of course," the doctor said.

Rose was semi-conscious as, mid-surgery, Chella explained a new strategy to the six female nurses she'd called in for support. Rose's uterus wasn't deflating, so the medical team inserted a balloon to help it safely contract down to size. Rose had no awareness of the balloon, but she did notice the local anesthesia was wearing off. She felt nauseous and light-headed, symptoms exacerbated by an empty stomach.

"Gently push on her belly every few minutes and monitor the

blood flow, okay?" The nurses nodded, and Chella waved to Rose and Patrick as she left the operating room.

Rose flinched as a nurse pressed her palm into her paunch.

"Oh my gosh! She's bleeding!" someone shouted. In a scene reminiscent of *The Shining*, blood gushed from Rose's body. After hearing the dense splash on the floor, she passed out.

Rose came to, gagging, as nurses pumped her with morphine and blood thickener. Amidst a dozen cycles of conking out, waking up, and gagging, She looked to Patrick—totally pale, the blood drained from his face—and whispered, "Don't go."

Each time a nurse touched her tender midsection, more blood surged.

"Maybe it's the morphine," Patrick suggested to the head nurse. "See how she's choking and trying to throw up?"

Rose next awoke when her doctor rushed into the room and yelled at the nurses, "Stop! Everyone out!"

When the room was clear, Chella explained that Rose's uterus wasn't contracting and they'd have to keep her overnight to monitor the blood loss. Rose consented from her panicked fog, then slept through the night. Patrick went home to be with the kids, and Rose's mother joined her at the hospital.

By morning, nurses had given Rose four bags of blood to stabilize her.

"Looks like that's the end of the bleeding," a resident greeted her. "How are you feeling?"

"Better," Rose said, her body still weak.

"We'll just do a little ultrasound." He cleared his throat. "See what's going on in there."

"Since I'm not bleeding anymore, I can go home, right?" Rose sensed fear in the room, but was growing impatient. She wanted to be home with her boys.

"Actually," Chella said, "the fact that you're not bleeding is bad, considering what happened yesterday, so let's take a look."

The doctor pulled up the image—and burst into tears. Rose's uterus was on the brink of rupturing. Between the scars of her previous Cesareans and the balloon insertion, the excessive bleeding had stretched it to capacity.

"Rose, we can't give you any more blood. Your body can't process it," Chella said between tears. "If you continue to lose blood, you won't live for very long."

The doctor and her assistant explained that, if left alone, Rose's uterus would rupture and she'd die. But if they removed the balloon, they feared continued blood loss and possible death.

"My doctors just cried, tears streaming, trying to hold it back," Rose recalled. "When people are upset, I usually shut off so I can care for them." So she did; she comforted the doctors.

"Ladies," she said, "I love you. We're fine. My sons really need me. We'll be okay!"

I smiled. "So you're literally on your deathbed, caring for your own doctors?"

Rose shook her head, laughing. "I know, it's ridiculous."

While the team consulted with specialists, Rose began making calls and saying her good-byes. She understood this was the end. She called Patrick and heard her sons' sweet voices, then rang her father and told him she loved him. Her mother excused herself to have a cigarette outside, her face as white as the hospital sheets. When she returned and asked how Rose was doing, her daughter said, "Great!" She felt terrified that Rose had accepted her fate.

The doctors decided on a uterine fibroid embolization—cauterizing an artery through the groin to stop the bleeding—after which they would remove the balloon. If that failed, they'd do a hysterectomy, which they feared Rose wouldn't survive.

"I'd already gone to a place of acceptance," Rose shared with me. "If they'd told me, 'We're gonna dress like Bert and Ernie from

Sesame Street, do a happy dance, and you'll be good,' I probably would've said, 'Awesome!'"

Patrick got to the hospital as the doctors wheeled in Rose for the embolization. He showered her with kisses and told her he'd always love her while the anesthesiologist prepared her dose.

"Please make sure it's enough," she begged the doctor.

Though he reassured her, Rose was conscious for more than half the procedure. She smelled her burning flesh and heard the whirring of surgical tools. When the doctors shifted her body to remove the balloon, her brain flashed white with the worst pain of her life. In her head she screamed over and over for them to stop the surgery, but a nurse later told her all they heard were faint moans. The doctors were so focused on stabilizing her that they raced on, administering more anesthesia only toward the end.

When Rose came to and learned the operation was a success, she felt an overwhelming sense of joy and connection. She had endured, even if her baby hadn't.

The couple decided to name their lost son Ethan, for his strong heart.

"What makes my situation different from just having the miscarriage several years before is that sense of oneness, of love." Rose's eyes welled up. "I knew that Ethan wasn't really gone," she said, placing her hand over her heart.

During her hospital stay over the next four days, Rose had a chilling exchange with an attending nurse.

"I was so sensitive and raw, I could feel this energy from her, this hatred, like she didn't want to help me," she recalled. She was convinced the nurse had seen the late-term abortion in her file and assumed her patient had wanted it. Hoping to dispel the tension, she shared that she had just lost a son she longed for—that she'd been forced to terminate through a surgery that had nearly cost her her life. Immediately, Rose felt the energy shift; from that moment forward, the nurse engaged her with compassion.

"I was relieved she'd softened, but she shouldn't have treated me any differently from someone choosing to end a pregnancy," Rose decried. "There's such a stigma around abortion!"

I was saddened to hear how, from Rose's perspective, the nurse's ideology prevented her from providing quality care. It was yet another example that women who suffer pregnancy loss are disregarded, thrown away. Moreover, the stigma and judgment can compound the sense of shame already burdening many such women.

Rose's recovery from this ordeal stretched over two years. She was often disoriented and experienced severe short-term memory loss that required extra patience and support from Patrick and her mother.

Once the brain fog cleared, Rose grieved more consciously for Ethan.

"I was immensely grateful to be alive," Rose said. "Only later would I wish Ethan was there. Seeing other kids, thinking, 'Gosh, that's how old he would be . . . but I'm alive! Just be grateful for that.' I kept forcing positivity onto it."

Rose and Patrick intended to find a way to honor the loss more formally, though they hadn't planned anything specific yet.

"You deal with the immediate crisis, then you keep going." Rose sighed. "Socially, there isn't an acknowledgement of loss . . . though I think it's getting better."

When I pressed her to enumerate those improvements, she mentioned social media, but then dismissed it as shallow.

I asked her if she had any advice or self-care tips for others experiencing pregnancy loss.

"Self-care tips?" Rose shook her head. "We can get those anywhere. It's the emotional and spiritual self that needs reassurance."

I recalled my darkest hours of grieving, when I uncovered a source of strength, yet unravaged by pain and sadness, that convinced me I would overcome my loss and help others through theirs.

Rose's trajectory had been changed by her losses, too. Through them, she discovered a passion for using her energetic awareness for healing, which led her to study energy work. Now she enjoyed a fulfilling career she couldn't have imagined before Ethan entered her life.

After we'd said our good-byes, I sat with Rose's grief and reflected on my own. A nagging sensation wore on me as I unpacked what I was coming to see as a glorification of pregnancy. For Rose, as for Katie and others, being pregnant was anything but sexy or romantic; in fact, it posed grave risks to both mother and child. My sense of womanhood began to disentangle itself from motherhood and its initial hallmark of pregnancy.

I knew my grief would entail further unraveling and acceptance.

Rose's final kernel of wisdom resounded in my head: "Be present with your grief, despite the pain. It's the only way through," she said, recalling Robert Frost's "the best way out is always through."

CHAPTER 17

Janice

"The assumption is pregnancy."

"HELLO!" JANICE BELLOWED as she stepped into the tidy apartment, and dropped her luggage with a satisfying whump on the narrow corridor's floor. "Oops, I mean, *Ni hao!*"

Lily's boyfriend, Alex, greeted Janice with a bear hug. "So nice to see you!" Alex pulled back to take in his guest: sultry, if tired, brown eyes, warm-umber complexion, broad-lipped smile, and thick, dark hair combed into a prim bun, sporting small gold hoops, urban-chic black duds accentuated with a colorful floral scarf, and black boots. "How was the flight?"

Before she could answer, Alex raised an eyebrow at Janice's small duffel.

"Oh, please!" Janice said with a smile. "You know I travel light."

They laughed and made small talk as Alex carried her bag into the sunlit living room.

Janice plopped down on the pristine white sofa, where she hoped to rest for a few hours before Lily returned from the office. The two women hadn't caught up in ages, and Janice knew her friend would insist on showing her all the latest bars in the bustling Shanghai neighborhood.

The sofa was a welcoming cloud of comfort after the trafficky cab rides and packed flight. Janice didn't remember the furniture from her last visit; the place was tiny but decorated just so—another mark of poshness creeping into their mid-thirties existence.

"God, I feel awful." Janice winced at the brightness of the room, her stomach tight with cramps. She'd just flown twelve hours from her home in London. *Bloody airplane food.* She dismissed her discomfort. "Enough about me and my whinging!"

They talked for an hour before Alex headed back to work downtown. Janice waved good-bye from the sofa, then got up to use the bathroom. She nearly tripped over her feet when she noticed a poppy-red pool soaking into the once virgin-white cushion she'd just been sitting on.

"Shit!" she gasped, entranced by the horrific stain.

She pulled off her jeans and underwear—now a plastered mess—tossed them into the bathtub, and fished out fresh underpants and the only menstrual pad from her bag. Mostly clothed again, she grabbed a kitchen brush from under the sink and a salad bowl from the dishrack, filled the bowl with soapy water, and—thus armed with supplies to help her avoid broaching this embarrassing incident with her hosts—scurried back to the living room.

"Shit!" she cried, louder now, scrubbing and rinsing and scrubbing harder, exerting a formidable amount of energy for her travel-weary body. She scoured the cushion for an hour, until the last drop of blood was gone—at which point she let out a sigh of relief, grateful for the cleanability of modern fabrics.

She blasted the wet cushion with a hairdryer from her perch on the other side of the sofa as she plotted her next moves.

"I went out to find sanitary towels," Janice told me in her dazzling British accent as she held a cup of tea in the noisy brunch spot where we'd met to talk, conveniently located near the podcasting conference that had brought her to San Francisco. "But I didn't know the language. So that was . . . fun," she said sarcastically, with a tilt of her head.

"Tell me more about the sanitary pad issue," I implored, breaking off a piece of the cafe's famous "millionaire's bacon" she'd insisted I try. I felt myself blush, recalling both my strong aversion to wearing pads and my ignorance that wearing tampons may not have been the most efficient, or the safest, approach during a miscarriage. "Was a certain product not available there, or was it more of a language or cultural barrier finding them . . . ?"

"All of the above. They didn't have the ones I'm used to. Actually, the best I've found were in Korea," she explained, with a *Who knew?* shrug.

Janice, now thirty-nine, travels frequently for work and pleasure; she's a true nomad in spirit, a podcaster/business coach by profession. "Luckily, you can point"—she gestured to her crotch— "or dig up something in the supermarket that does the job, so I was fine."

By the time Alex returned from work, Janice was lounging on the sofa as if nothing had happened. She still felt off, with persistent cramping, but it was nothing, she figured, that an Advil or two couldn't tackle.

When Lily arrived home shortly after Alex, however, Janice realized she'd soaked through a heavy-duty pad in less than two hours.

"I just thought it was an unusually heavy period, changed my pad, and dealt with the cramping," she said. "I chalked it up to jet lag and possibly a stomach bug."

The cramping and bleeding, punctuated by thick blood clots, lasted three days and put a damper on her China trip. Janice had been on birth control since she was fifteen. She'd never wanted kids and certainly hadn't tried to conceive, so the thought of pregnancy or miscarriage never crossed her mind.

"Didn't think anything of it!" Janice said. "Fast-forward a few months, when my periods were normal again, I read something online about miscarriages, and—'Oh, oh, oh shiiit . . . yes, of course!'"

Soon after reading the article, Janice visited her doctor friend in Canada and told him about her experience in Shanghai. Initially, he was shocked to hear that she hadn't understood it was a miscarriage, but slightly less so when he learned she'd been taking oral contraceptives for two decades to manage heavy periods.

"Wow, what are the chances that birth control wouldn't work?" I was too stunned to filter my astonishment.

"I don't even *see* my boyfriend that often!" Janice said, her face screwed into an expression of disbelief.

Janice estimated she was only a few weeks pregnant when the miscarriage took place. When I asked if she'd experienced any pregnancy symptoms, she flashed me a big smile.

"Nope, my body did good!" She laughed heartily. "It knew! 'You don't want kids? I got you.' Whew!" She sighed theatrically. "I didn't know I had miscarried until it was far too late. I didn't receive any of the care you're supposed to because I was clueless."

"What kind of care?" I asked.

"Well, a doctor's supposed to check that everything is cleared out. Otherwise, there's a cancer risk." Janice scrunched up her nose. "You know, leftover baby's in there, just hanging out, like, blech!" She relaxed her face and lowered her voice. "I should've gotten an ultrasound and checked that everything was flushed out, working, and back to normal."

Janice's story shocked me on multiple levels. She had diligently used contraception yet had still gotten pregnant—that rare case of the pill not being effective that I'd only read about in the fine print on posters in my Ob/Gyn's office. Furthermore, here was a woman my age who'd never wanted children and was seemingly happy childfree and in a committed relationship spanning over six years. She and her boyfriend, Gareth, lived in separate countries but still managed to cultivate a fulfilling partnership. Was she real? Were she and Gareth, five years her junior, really at peace with a childfree relationship?

Curious about Janice's take on family, I inquired about her upbringing.

"I have no family; I was adopted and it was a shit show," Janice said with a cheeriness that seemed either forced or performative, I couldn't yet tell. "A lot of people say, 'Oh no, you poor thing!' But no family? It's awesome!"

With so much instability and uncertainty growing up in foster care, Janice learned at a young age to fend for herself. She worked in human resources, started several businesses, and eventually found her way to coaching. Given her gregarious, humorous nature, I was surprised to hear that her career centered on supporting introverts. Did she consider herself one?

Yes, she said, thanks to her upbringing—always the feeling of being in the shadows.

Janice married "young," in her mid-twenties, and both she and her ex-husband were firm about not wanting children throughout their ten years together.

I wanted to know how Janice had discussed the miscarriage with Gareth. Did he harbor any feelings about it?

"At first, I didn't even tell my boyfriend," Janice said. "But then I thought, *He kind of has a right to know.* But telling him took some doing." She sipped on her tea, her gaze lingering in the steaming cup. "There's never a right time to tell someone. Normally, we're working, or we might be out to dinner. When's a 'good' time? 'Hey, let's go to the park!'—but then, 'Why the hell are we going to the park?'"

Janice told Gareth when they next saw each other—at a park.

"Because he's younger than me by five years—although since he's a guy, it's more like ten!" Janice's giggle was irresistible. "I've always said, 'If you want kids, exit stage left. I'm *not* going to change my mind.' So when I told him, I was wondering how he'd react because that would be a telltale sign if he actually wanted kids."

After Janice explained what happened, she took Gareth's hand and asked him, straight faced, "Are you okay?"

"Yeah, I'm good." Gareth squeezed her hand and gave her a wink as they continued strolling among the sycamore trees.

"Yeah?" She stopped and looked him in the eyes.

He nodded with a reassuring smile.

"Okay, good," she said, relieved.

I recalled several nature walks with my husband, Joe, in the years between fertility clinic visits and the big miscarriage, when we'd revisit the topic of children, mutually making sure the other was okay with status quo—i.e., no longer pursuing having children. "Are you sure you won't be disappointed or resentful down the road?" I'd ask. After Joe patiently assured me he'd still love me and we'd have a fulfilling life together without children—and that we could always adopt later on—I'd usually end up in tears, relieved, and needing his embrace. We would be okay, his arms told me; we alone would be enough. *I* was enough, just as Kari's husband had expressed to her. I didn't have to hold that burden in my marriage—at least, not anymore.

But the miscarriage shook everything up for me, throwing my— even Joe's—resolve into momentary doubt. Now that we knew I could get pregnant, were we certain remaining childfree was the right decision?

I asked Janice if she ever felt a speck of doubt after she realized she'd lost a pregnancy.

"Yes, actually, there was one moment," Janice admitted, looking into my eyes. "In the shower, after talking to my doctor friend, absorbing that I had been pregnant, that I could even *get* pregnant. For a split second, I asked myself if I'd have wanted a kid." She paused, her lips opening into a smile. "Then: *Wake up, Janice!* I just needed to be more aware of what was going on with my body."

"So, even though you were adamant about not wanting a kid, you still considered how you'd have felt had the pregnancy been viable?" Had I reached my limit of comprehension, even empathy? Janice was so solid about not wanting kids, and still certain now that she didn't want kids. Had it truly been a moment of doubt about her path, or had it just been a fleeting thought, that *What if . . .?* And what difference did it make?

My stuckness glared at me like a hangnail caught on a delicate knit sweater.

"Right. What would've happened if my body hadn't gotten rid of it? How would I feel about it then?"

Janice nodded and I felt my shoulders drop with the validation that she, too, had her doubts.

"But, mainly, it was understanding that I needed to pay more attention to my body and the signs it was giving me," she clarified. "Perhaps there were other signs I didn't notice. It was in combination with so many other things . . ."

"Like traveling?" I suggested. "That can really throw the body off."

"Absolutely!"

I asked how the miscarriage changed Janice's relationship to her body. Was she more in tune with it now?

"Luckily, I discovered the [menstrual] cup. When you bleed in a sanitary napkin—and FYI, I don't do tampons—you don't get a sense of the color or viscosity or anything of that nature, which tells you a lot about your health. So the cup is awesome." Janice cackled. "Not great for flying, though, because suction *is* a factor, and people don't tell you that!"

She expounded on the importance of women not only paying more attention to their bodies, particularly as they get older, but also sharing their wisdom with one another. "Our minds and bodies are constantly changing, and changing regardless of whether we want them to!" she said. "But people don't talk about it. Honestly, I don't know many women who've been through miscarriage—that I'm aware of. More women have told me about their sexual assault or rape experiences. Yet there's not enough women talking about any of these issues!"

"All common experiences, unfortunately," I said.

"*Very* common experiences," she corrected. "Also, lots of women may have had miscarriages and, like me, not have known."

Janice feels an overall lack of sex education, and the poor quality of the little there is, are to blame for under-recognition of early pregnancy loss as well as ignorance of miscarriage symptoms and best-care practices.

"Sex ed teaches you about periods, intercourse, safe sex, pregnancy—IF you get any of that! You might even learn a bit about abortion, depending on where you are, but that's a big *if.*"

Janice currently lives in Mexico, a largely Catholic nation where, in her friends' experiences, society—including many doctors—frowns upon abortion. Since medical procedures for miscarriage are identical to those for abortion, miscarriage procedures and those receiving or performing them bore a similar stigma.

"It's assumed that women will get pregnant, then it's assumed that they will go to term." Janice wasn't just referring to Mexico, but of the lasting worldview of women's roles as mothers; or rather, successful mothers. "The assumption is pregnancy because *baby equals happy*, which may be the case, but people don't think about what happens when a pregnancy doesn't pan out."

As someone who's staunchly uninterested in becoming a mother but relishes being "the cool auntie" to friends' children, Janice spoke directly to the dangers of pronatalism, the belief that childbearing and parenthood are desirable for social reasons as well as the proliferation of the human species. Echoing Noreen's lamentations that women feel undue pressure to procreate, Janice complained that omnipresent pronatalist attitudes made women who choose childfree lives feel inadequate.

"This imperative of 'I'm a woman, so I must have kids because that proves I'm a value to society'—it's crazy!" Janice said, wildly stirring a spoon in her cup. "Not only that, the statistics of women who die during childbirth, especially in the United States, are ridiculous!"

I couldn't argue with that. Maternal mortality statistics are indeed startling, especially for Black, Indigenous, and women of color: overall, seventeen maternal deaths for every 100,000 births in the US, the highest rate of any developed country; and Black women suffer maternal death at over twice that rate.[16]

Janice's frustration over pronatalism extended to insurance. With her frequent travel, she had arranged for global healthcare rather than the basic travel insurance one might procure for an international vacation. She wanted the comprehensive coverage, but was annoyed that perinatal care couldn't be deselected from her package.

"They refused, point blank, to take out the maternity care stuff, so now I have to pay more for it," Janice kvetched—meaning, pay more than a man would. "Even if I'd had a hysterectomy and couldn't physically have kids, as a woman, I still have to pay for it." She held a palm up in the air and let her jaw hang slack for effect. "But, I suppose that's a different topic . . ."

"Oh, don't get me started on sales tax on tampons!" I said, smiling, as she let out a peal of laughter.

She was quick to add that she felt nervous discussing pronatalism with such negatively charged emotion, as she empathized deeply with women who felt called to motherhood yet struggled with infertility and pregnancy loss.

"There are so many different facets, but at the end of the day we're all just human," she said. "As long as you're a good human, that's all that should matter."

Janice's miscarriage not only brought her greater self-awareness, it also allowed her to support her close friend, Victoria, through the pains and uncertainties of her own pregnancy loss. After Victoria's abortion with mifepristone and misoprostol—the pills generally prescribed to miscarrying women to induce labor and clear out the uterus—Janice shared some of what she had experienced and read about to help Victoria know what to expect. She warned her about the cramping—"You may become friends with your toilet"—and described the thick clotting, heavy bleeding, and days of recovery that, for women farther along in their pregnancy, could last for several weeks.

Victoria thanked Janice. "I never would've known any of this," she told her. Her doctor hadn't informed her, and she couldn't find any resources online.

"Abortion is just like miscarriage—the same physical and often emotional experiences, the exact same procedures," Janice told me. While the former remains more stigmatized and politicized than the latter, she said, both are taboo.

First Rose and now Janice had each drawn connections between abortion and miscarriage, stigma and compassion. Both had expressed the importance of sharing our stories of loss to support others, but also to cultivate more compassion for women in general— for example, amongst healthcare workers.

It dawned on me that a friend of mine likely wouldn't have opened up to me about her recent abortion had she not known that I was writing about pregnancy loss. While she had felt it was the right decision, she wasn't comfortable talking about it with close friends or family. She wrestled with her sadness and disconnection as she grieved the child she wasn't yet ready to raise.

Janice felt that the lack of information about pregnancy loss— whether the loss is intended or not—begets misinformation, which in turn begets feelings of guilt and shame.

"We scrutinize the woman," she nearly howled. "'I was sleeping on the wrong side of the bed,' or 'I didn't feng shui my house properly.'" Her jokey smile flickered out. "That guilt can be crushing! It can destroy a relationship! Plus, there's no time off for it in the workplace, especially in America." She shook her head. "You guys don't get time off for anything!"

Salaried parents generally receive time off to pick up children from school or tend to a child's illness, she said, so why not extend that courtesy to workers who experience pregnancy loss? "No questions asked, and it shouldn't count toward paid time off!" she cried. "As someone who's worked in HR, you should just be able to say, 'I need some time off.' Period. End of story."

Janice kept steering the conversation away from herself and toward the larger plight of women, particularly those who've suffered pregnancy loss and wish they'd been better treated and/or informed. Was this tendency an inevitability of interviewing someone who never wanted children, or was there something deeper? I persevered, wanting to know more about her personal experience.

"What did you learn about yourself through the miscarriage?" I asked.

"Confirmed I don't want kids! Confirmed my partner doesn't want kids!" she said, smiling. "But I also know people change, so every six months or so I'll ask Gareth, 'You still sure about this?'"

Janice confessed to taking Gareth to see friends who have adorable kids just to make sure he was absolutely certain. He's always reassured her that he's happier without children.

"I'm lucky, because I know the older you get, some people realize they actually want—even need—kids," Janice said. "That's why I continue to check in."

She said she rarely brings up her miscarriage unprompted—i.e., not in the presence of someone experiencing pregnancy loss. Most friends and colleagues aren't aware of her loss, and she's happy to keep it that way unless she thinks it might support someone's healing.

"It always brings up questions. The fact that my best friend asked, 'So, you want kids now?' Ugh," she groaned with a sly grin.

I took in Janice's comedic sigh with a sense of relief. Loss is complicated, whether we deeply desired that thing we lost or never wanted it in the first place. And it's okay for it to be complicated—messy, paradoxical, confusing. It's okay to want or not to want, to grieve intensely or to find the dark humor, if that's available to us. Janice's story gave me permission to feel less like a pariah for my ambivalence about having kids. She reminded me that I'm human, and that is, or at least should be, enough.

Obviously, Janice is the cool auntie.

CHAPTER 18

K T

"The world needs our love!"

FROM THE MOMENT I MET HER, with her long, flowing clothes, earth tones, and shoulder-length, gray-golden hair tied loosely in a bun, KT exuded warmth. She had just come from the YMCA and was ordering juice and a bagel. We found a quiet table in the cafe to chat. Her voice was as soothing and reassuring as her soft features: a gentle smile and bright eyes. This woman was very much alive and present, quietly comfortable in her own skin.

Raised in a liberal, upper-middle-class family, KT dropped out of Oberlin College as a young woman and moved to San Francisco with her now-husband, Doug, to become a professional dancer. That's where the symptoms first began.

In 1978, when KT was twenty-three years old, she fell mysteriously ill. An otherwise healthy woman, she developed peritonitis, an inflammation of the lining of the abdominal and pelvic cavity, as well as infections in her diaphragm, liver, spleen, ovaries, uterus, and intestines. She was dying, and no one understood why. The best the doctors could do was give her a general antibiotic to curb the presenting infections.

"My gynecologist could not for the life of her figure out what I had," KT told me, her kind eyes acknowledging my bewilderment.

KT continued to work despite the pain she felt throughout her body. Wherever her dance troupe toured, she would locate a new clinic in the hopes of finding someone who could treat her.

"In Vancouver, dancing, I thought the music was going faster than it was," she told me, shaking her head. "I was really not well. I went to a clinic and they said, 'Oh, *we* know what you have. You have PID!' They knew because they have socialized medicine and this was a disease that prostitutes get." She laughed quietly. "I had a working-class disease, but my middle-class gynecologist had never seen it." In that instance, KT realized that diseases, like people, were associated with class.

It was the onset of an epidemic of pelvic inflammatory disease (PID), when the first wave of middle-class women swapped out their fussier, calendar-sensitive oral contraceptives for the convenience of intrauterine devices (IUDs). Back in the 1970s, IUDs weren't tested for safety and effectiveness like they are today. Eventually, clinicians traced the growing outbreak to a poorly designed IUD called Dalkon Shield, whose manufacturer went bankrupt facing mounting lawsuits.

By today's standards, PID is both common and easily treatable. At the time, however, most medical practitioners weren't aware of it. KT was one of thousands of women to suffer from undiagnosed PID, although, coincidentally, she'd never even had an IUD. She likely got the disease during intercourse from contact with E. coli or some other common bacteria, which led to an infection that, left untreated, became life-threatening. Her symptoms went undiagnosed for two years before the clinic in Vancouver recognized the disease and finally gave her clarity.

The Vancouver team hospitalized KT and did exploratory surgery to understand the extent of the damage. They found her fallopian tubes were completely blocked with scar tissue and declared she would never bear children. They prescribed a rotating regimen of antibiotics and bed rest for six months.

"I wanted to be a professional," she said with a casual wave of her hand. "I never really thought about family." She paused. "I mean, it's a little disturbing that my body wasn't working, that the option was gone, but I grew up in a period where people had sex and tried not to have kids. So, it just relaxed something in us. Not that I didn't want kids, I just hadn't really thought about it."

KT spent several months out of work recovering at her mother's home in Los Angeles before heading back to San Francisco. Her doctor recommended rest and urged her to learn to live with the illness, whatever it was. After hearing that she would likely never dance again, KT looked beyond her doctor and Western medicine for help. She ended up seeking treatment from an acupuncturist and Chinese herbalist.

At last, she began to feel more like her old self. Living with PID, she had suffered excruciating menstrual pain. "My God!" she exclaimed, her eyes wide. "I never had bad periods before, but the scar tissue . . . It was a ton of pain!" Now she was able to get back to dancing and feeling good in her body.

Life was going fine, then one day, when KT was twenty-seven—"Oops! I'm pregnant!" she told me with a huge smile.

She and Doug had stopped using birth control, assuming that she was sterile. She was three months along when they found out. It was a total shock.

"There I was, at twenty-three, thinking I'm never going to be able to have a child, then twenty-seven and I'm pregnant!" She smiled to herself. "That was when Doug realized how much he'd wanted a kid."

The couple announced she was pregnant and decided to get married. "I came from that era where you just live with your person even if you were going to live with them for sixty years," she explained. But with a child on the way, marriage was the socially acceptable norm, even in their progressive artist circle. They planned a casual wedding for the following month—marriage at city hall and a party in Golden Gate Park with family and friends. "We were hippies," KT sighed more than spoke, an air of nostalgia in her voice.

She and Doug were living in Hunters Point, a low-income neighborhood in San Francisco, without health insurance at the time. When she was four months pregnant, she went to the local clinic for a sonogram. "It's not there anymore," the nurse told her. "There's no heartbeat. You'll need to get a D&C."

KT remembers little else from that visit.

Since her local clinic was unable to do the D&C, they referred her to one in Oakland; but instead of performing a D&C, the staff inserted little bamboo sticks into her cervix to force it gently open, told her she would naturally pass the fetus and wouldn't need the D&C, then sent her home.

KT had no idea what to expect for her impending miscarriage, the clinic having provided scant details, let alone a rough timeline.

"I mean, this is all I remember," she said. "They may have actually given me more information. I just don't know how cognizant I was. Doug probably should have been there with me, but, you know"—she grinned sheepishly—"*We're all independent.* That's how we saw ourselves in that era."

By the time KT got home, she had already started to miscarry.

"It was brutal!" she recalled, her mouth agape. "It happened over about twenty-four hours, but what's so interesting is that I had a mini experience of being in labor."

KT began having contractions and experienced more severe pain. It was around midnight when she finally asked Doug to drive her to the emergency room.

"Just as we got in the car, I said, 'I'm ready to throw up.' Then I went through transition, my water broke, and the fetus popped out in the car!"

Doug kept driving until they reached the hospital. Staff rushed to admit KT and confirm she was okay, then they presented her with the fetus.

"It was amazing to see," KT effused.

By the time the couple got back to their home in San Francisco, it was already dawn. And the day of their wedding.

KT laughed, thinking back on the whirlwind forty-eight hours. She and Doug disclosed the miscarriage to their close friends and family, who then passed the news on to everyone else.

"We were all artists and hippies," she said, smiling. "People said, 'Oh, well,' and, 'Hey, you don't have to get married now!' since so many of us only got married because we were pregnant."

I wanted to know how KT felt heading straight into her wedding coming off the miscarriage.

"All sorts of interesting pressure . . ."

"How did you experience that?" I asked.

"I was totally wiped out. I don't even know if I slept," she said. "I was really worried about whether I was making the right decision by getting married."

I was fairly taken aback hearing this. KT had already spoken so affectionately of Doug, it never crossed my mind that she would have doubted him or the relationship.

"We were getting married because we were pregnant, and then we were no longer pregnant. I wasn't sure why we were doing it. It even brings up the question of why we were getting married *because* we were pregnant." She leaned toward me, her head outstretched. "But it ended up being the biggest gift."

KT was elated about the marriage once they tied the knot. Within two weeks, something had unlocked within her, a certain appreciation of the life she and Doug were now creating together.

She imagined herself and Doug holding hands and walking together through life. Suddenly, she could discern the real value of marriage, which she hadn't previously considered.

Doug, meanwhile, was hit hard by the loss.

"He sobbed during that whole period where I lost the fetus. He really wanted a kid," KT said tenderly. "We got married April 10th, so by the end of that next September, 1983, we were pregnant with our son Haley."

I asked her how she felt about the loss.

"I went through so much around the PID. There was a lot of dis-sociation—from my body generally, but also from my reproductive body. My sister always had really bad cramps and endometriosis, whereas I always had my period for a day or two and danced through it. Then, boom, for my body to go through this trauma! I detached from myself with all that pain."

KT thought the earlier dissociation may have protected her from some of the physical and emotional pain of the miscarriage. She was quick to add that, above all, she felt gratitude for having gotten married.

I was curious if she or Doug carried any loss anxiety forward from the first pregnancy.

"No!" she cried. "I think because I grew up in a household where there was a lot of physical freedom. My mom was really active, and when we would fall, you would just get up and go! Nobody asked, 'Are you okay?' One of the things that Doug and I both agreed on is that the body does heal. It's an amazing thing." She shrugged. "I sort of took it as listening to my body."

When I asked if KT felt more in touch with her body during the pregnancy, she said certainly not in the first one.

"I'm a dancer, so I know my body well, and I'm used to controlling it. I think the thing about labor—both the miscarriage and the 'labor' labor—was, wow, this body knows something, and I have no say in it!"

KT and Doug went to brooding and breathing classes, but that all flew out the window during Haley's birth. "It was much more of an experience," KT explained. She was in the moment—letting her body be rather than exerting control over it.

What little she did recall about her body in the second pregnancy was positive.

"Loved it, loved it!" she boasted. She gushed about her pregnancy with Haley, punctuated with several "Oh my God!"s and light gasps verging on swooning.

She was thankful she hadn't had the D&C; that meant she knew what it meant to go through labor and was able to compare the first experience to her experience with Haley.

"Sometimes women's water breaks right away. Mine broke right after transition. And it had the same shape!" she said, her hands drawing squiggles in the air. "So I got a little rehearsal; I just didn't know it at the time."

As KT complained that so many women get disconnected from the beauty and wonder of their bodies through medication and surgery during labor, she suddenly recalled what Doug's mother had said to her when she miscarried: "Do you realize that 50 percent of pregnancies are miscarriages?"

Though the widely quoted statistics aren't quite so high for the general population now, nor were they then—the rate is closer to 25 percent, with increasing risk for older women—Doug's mother may well have experienced such high rates of loss within her own social network.

KT felt comforted to hear how common miscarriage was. "It helped me because I remember thinking, my body can't do this, I'm not good at this." Once she miscarried, KT stopped believing in the possibility of having children. In her mind, she kept hearing the doctors in Vancouver telling her she was sterile and thought, *My reproductive thing is not happening.*

"I didn't feel like I wasn't a woman," she clarified. "It just made me feel bad about myself. Like, I can't do this and most women can."

When I noted how common that refrain is among women who have miscarried, KT nodded with a deep frown. She expressed her gratitude for many of the older women in her life who reassured her that miscarriage is just something that happens. Her own mother had four miscarriages along with her four living children.

KT's birthing instructor had asked each of the women in her class what she feared most. "That I'll end up isolated in a suburb," KT answered. The instructor shared that she had two kids who she simply brought along with her when she traveled the globe. Hearing this alternative version of parenting shifted KT's perspective. She was able to see herself both as a professional dancer and a mother. She wouldn't have to give up one for the other.

When I asked about her experience of motherhood, she lit up and flashed a huge smile. "Ah, well, it never stops, and that just blows me away."

Her son, Haley, now thirty-five, and his wife, Jenny, have been trying to conceive for years, without success. KT empathizes and is supportive of them, though she still has mixed feelings about repro- duction. "It's sad for everybody and it's also okay," she said, nodding emphatically. "I worry about the population on the planet, and I don't believe anybody's one kid is going to be the savior of the world." When I smiled and raised an eyebrow, she softened her tone. "But it *is* sad."

Both Haley and Jenny are only children, and Haley's cousins are all much younger. There is the feeling that when Haley and Jenny die, assuming they don't end up with kids of their own, there won't be much of a family left. So KT and Haley discussed what that might mean.

"We have a very rigid society around parenthood," KT bemoaned with fiery eyes. "Why is *your* kid the only avenue for love and nurtur- ing? Why is that the ultimate heart opener? Why can't you help other people? Why can't you help someone else's kid?"

Doug encouraged Haley and Jenny to get involved in the lives of their friends who have children. KT acknowledged that Doug could neither design nor force that kind of relationship, but she hoped that by talking with them about the possibility of helping their friends' families, they might find greater purpose and a means to fulfill their desire for children.

KT's advice to other women and couples struggling with pregnancy loss and infertility was to consider offering their love in ways distinct from biological parenting.

"The world desperately needs our love to happen in other forms," she pleaded, her upper body hovering over the table with urgency. "One of the things that happens when you're a parent is your heart really opens up. But I don't believe that has to be limited to your own kid. As a parent, your ego gets caught up in how your kid unfolds, which is the worst thing for that kid! And most parents don't see it."

She argued that it might be easier for people to let go of their ego if they loved something that wasn't their own child. She suggested it might even be a purer kind of love. "Our society has put so much pressure on the couple, and it's just too much!" she said, shaking her head. "People need to extend their notion of family beyond the biological family. We're going to need it more and more as the world unfolds. But we don't have a lot of skills toward that."

By the end of our conversation about expanding our concept of love and building community, I was fantasizing about adopting this woman as a mother. In fact, several times, I heard my own mother's voice in KT: "It might not be the best thing that your kid learns to read at four. That kid may just need to wander in the dirt and pick flowers and eat them until they're seven!"

I suppose I have a thing for opinionated hippie moms . . . but also for women who embrace the nearly implausible, somewhat terrifying notion that I can have a deeply fulfilling life without children.

CHAPTER 19

Golda

"I love being a woman."

GOLDA'S CONTRACTIONS HAD ALREADY STARTED when she left the doctor's office. Her partner, Max, raced out of work to meet her, along with the midwife and doula, at the couple's beach bungalow in San Diego, California.

The midwife laid a plastic covering over the bed and piled on fluffy pillows and cotton towels while the doula drew a warm bath and called Golda's acupuncturist. The birthing Dream Team would support Golda through the next six hours of labor and delivery.

Golda, then a thirty-six-year-old children's yoga instructor, wondered about the duration and mechanics of labor, the baby's sex, and her pain tolerance. How big would the baby be?

In the end, her maternal instincts guided her without her ever needing to ask the Dream Team questions. At times she was in the tub, then on a giant yoga ball, now lying on the bed. She was awed that her body knew exactly what to do—what she was called to do. This was the power of mothering, of being a woman.

The acupuncturist, who'd been working with Golda for anxiety and depression, approached her on the bed and placed three needles in her toes. Immediately, Golda felt the baby descend. Minutes later, the midwife clipped the umbilical cord and placed the glistening baby boy in her trembling hands.

Tears streamed down Golda's flushed cheeks as she beheld the lifeless creature in her palm. Baby Truman looked fully developed, with a button nose, doll's ears and eyes, and miniature arms and legs. Yet, the ultrasound that morning had confirmed what she'd already learned earlier in the week from the midwife: the nearly twenty-week-old fetus's heart had stopped beating. Nobody knew why.

As Golda and her Dream Team waited for the placenta to come through, quiet sadness in the room turned to concern for the mother's health. Golda's contractions had stopped, but the midwife was unable to obtain the remaining placenta. Golda was quickly losing blood.

"We need to get you to a hospital," the midwife announced.

Within the hour, Golda was in an ambulance headed to the ER, where the issue was swiftly resolved. Max took her home that evening, and she recovered over the next weeks in the company of friends and natural healers.

Golda acknowledged to me that her professional perinatal support, largely removed from mainstream Western medical care, was a luxury most women and families in the US could not afford. Yet her experience of pregnancy loss shared many of the hallmark features of grief and loneliness, transformation of the intimate-partner relationship, and reckoning with a higher power and oneself.

"Tru's birth was so beautiful . . . and so devastating," she said, breaking into a full-body sob. I handed her a box of tissues from the credenza behind her couch, where we sat in her peaceful, minimalist Oakland apartment. I reached for my herbal tea to quell the sisterly urge to hug my host. Connected with one another by a mutual friend and former yoga colleague, this was the first time we'd met, and although I believed she would welcome the soothing gesture, I felt I needed to keep my composure.

"I held both of those tensions," Golda whispered. "It was so incredible to deliver him and be at home with support. But then not to have this life we'd been planning . . . How do you restructure? It was all so confusing."

Golda and Max placed Truman in a small wooden box lined with tissue paper, then arranged his body in a goddess pose—feet together, knees apart, hands on his heart. They buried him under the canopy of a giant, windswept cypress overlooking the Pacific, a sacred site they had hiked by a handful of times in their seven months together.

Days later, Golda passed a twin fetus the size of an olive. The doctor had mentioned the possibility of twins during the ultrasound. Truman's sibling must have perished in her womb much earlier in the pregnancy. Golda flushed it down the toilet where she'd discovered it, her body aching with grief.

"That whole week, time stood still," Golda, now forty-five, recalled, her short brunette curls lifting with each heaving cry. "I couldn't understand how one day I was carrying a healthy baby, then all of a sudden, halfway through my pregnancy, everything changed. It's life and death, within seconds. The baby is here and then it's not. I may never understand it."

After the loss, Max took a week off work to be by Golda's side and welcome the many friends and relatives who brought them meals and mourned with them. Golda had only dated Max for two months before she got pregnant. They'd fallen fast and hard for each other. During the pregnancy, as Golda struggled with preexisting depression and hormones flooded her body and mind, she'd faced growing doubts about the relationship. She wanted the child, she was certain, but it wasn't clear to her whether Max was the right fit.

To her surprise, the relationship blossomed as they mourned together for Truman. Whenever she thought she'd cried herself out, more tears would come. She was exhausted by the loss, her keening, and the physical discomfort. Yet Max held her through the pain and suffering. He helped her accept the loss.

"I was pissed at God for taking away the plan that God had given me to begin with," Golda told me. "My partner, though, came from a place of trusting that the loss was God's way for us. I couldn't see it then, but he helped me understand that it was God's will, which I found extremely helpful. It really brought us together."

Golda grew up in a liberal Jewish household and lives a deeply spiritual life grounded in her faith. She recently chose to start using her Hebrew name as well as her birth name, Jodi. Her yoga teaching enterprise is a natural extension of her spirituality and life philosophy.

"I really believe there's this divine orchestration that is happening for us all," Golda explained in a near-whisper, her wide eyes aglow with wonder. "Those moments when my partner offered that perspective of surrender to me, I felt a deep sense of peace and trust. It's so tender, though. I probably needed to hear it from him at that very moment: *I* didn't will it, but God did."

With Golda's anxiety and hormones still surging after the delivery, Max offered to cancel the wedding they'd planned. *I'm going to super-mom it*, Golda thought. In the throes of her grief, just six weeks after the loss, she went with Max and their immediate families to Sedona for an intimate ceremony. The marriage wasn't legal, and perhaps that was for the best. It was, Golda said, a challenging relationship.

"In my woo-woo mind," Golda said with a roll of her eyes, "I feel like Truman knew that our relationship wasn't the one for him to come into. As devastating as it is to have lost him, I really believe that he chose to leave us. And I find peace in that."

I was struck by Golda's profound calm and confidence. Her inner strength extended outward to her muscular frame, long, toned arms, and graceful posture, her legs tucked delicately beneath her sculpted torso and wide bosom, all of it accentuated by form-fitting activewear.

Her eyes were deep wells of knowing, self-knowledge, and her full lips rested in a placid quarter-smile.

I heard the familiar echo of Molly's story in Golda's. *The baby I lost knew it wasn't the right partner.* I recognized the comfort it gave those women to make the connection between the dual losses of their pregnancy and their life partners. Others I spoke to, like Jackie, felt affirmed by their successful pregnancies: *The baby will come with the right partner, at the right time.* Yet far more women suffer losses despite being in loving, committed relationships. There is no rule, no one-size-fits-all. Infinite paths to healing and acceptance abound. It's up to each of us to find our respective path and embark on that journey.

For Golda, locating her path meant taking six months off from teaching to process the loss and find her bearings. The sight of mothers with strollers or holding a child's hand crossing the street would send her into crying spells. She needed to prepare herself mentally for working with children again. What would she say?

Her fear of judgment dissolved into excitement to see her students.

"Did you have your baby?" an eight-year-old girl asked, pointing to Golda's flat belly.

"What's its name?" another girl shouted, sashaying across the gym floor. "Can you show us pictures?"

Golda drew a deep breath, as second and third graders in sweats and leggings gathered around her.

"Okay, everyone, let's get on our mats and into a comfortable lotus pose, hands at our sides." Golda sat with her legs crossed, modeling her instructions, as the children spread out across the worn wood floor. "Good. Now I know you're all curious about where I've been, so I'm going to share something with you that's very close to my heart. Do you think we can all sit still for a moment and listen?"

The children hung on to Golda's every word as she told them about her initial excitement of her pregnancy, then the loss and sadness.

Some students cried; others asked questions, which Golda answered as openly and age-appropriately as she could.

"I took the risk of sharing my truth and trusted that parents and the school would be okay with it," Golda told me, breaking into a grin. "They were all so great about it!"

I asked Golda if she wanted to try conceiving again. Was there an unfulfilled desire to have a child?

"No, not with him," she said. "That relationship was super challenging."

Golda had always wanted to be a mom with a large brood: a set of twins, a few adoptees, and at least one child with special needs. She'd worked with kids her whole life and appreciated the range of challenges and personalities. Her grandmother was a twin, and she was positive she would bear twins too.

After separating from Max, Golda approached dating with a clear agenda: she wanted kids and was looking for a committed father.

When she was forty, Golda briefly dated someone she adored but who expressed a hard "no" to having kids. He told her she was great, but that they were on a different trajectory of life; he wasn't interested in parenting.

Though Golda was initially heartbroken, as she sat with the pain and rejection, she realized she didn't actually want to be a mom.

"My whole life I had been so conditioned and programmed to think that this is what I wanted and what I'm supposed to do: get married, have kids, give my parents grandkids." Golda smiled serenely. "All of a sudden, by dating this man and hearing we weren't on the same path, I got really clear."

"And it wasn't about your feelings for him?" I asked.

"No, no, no, not at all," Golda said. "He's since passed away, but I'm so grateful to him for allowing me to see that parenting was not what I wanted."

Golda wrestled with how to share her new perspective with her family. She felt the news would come as a disappointment to her parents, who had always wanted more grandchildren, and to her older siblings, who wanted more cousins for their children. She dreaded the conversation with her parents, but their support triumphed. "This is your life," they told her; thankfully, they already had two grandkids. When she told her brothers and sisters-in-law that she felt selfish not having kids, they told her it would actually be more selfish of her to have a kid and not be a full "yes."

I couldn't overlook the parallels between Golda and me. We're both the youngest of the family, each with two older brothers who have kids, and we share a Jewish upbringing with expectations of bearing children. We've both squirmed with guilt for deciding to be childfree.

"You use the word *selfish*," I said, "which has come up so many times in my own thinking about not having kids. Hearing you express it now, I regret that it's been in my vocabulary. And yet the feeling is real."

Golda perked up. "Yes! It's a lot."

"I wonder how we unpack those feelings of selfishness and guilt," I mused.

"We have a similar cultural background and ancestry, but how much of that is even ours?" Golda wondered. "I can't tell you how powerful that guilt is. I can still hear my mother saying, 'Get married and have kids already, would you?'"

She explained that those negative feelings extend beyond the long-assumed and expressed family pressure to procreate.

"I truly experienced deep grief, sadness, and anger; that was very real for me then," she said. "But nearly ten years later, believing that loss was supposed to happen, I have a certain amount of guilt and even shame." She looked out the window as she gracefully shifted her legs beneath her. "Maybe it's about the collective women who miscarry. So many women who try and try and still . . ."

"Guilt because you've moved on from it?" I asked.

"Exactly." Golda's creased forehead softened as she smiled. "I'd love to hear your story, if you're open to sharing with me."

I indulged Golda with a condensed version of the fertility roller coaster, ambivalence around motherhood, trying and wanting to have a kid, then getting surprisingly close, only to lose my pregnancy, my hope, and my confidence. How I now wondered, *What do I want, and how can I be sure anymore?*

I, too, felt the guilt of having found peace with both my loss and choosing a childfree life, especially in the context of writing this book. I was and remain fearful of offending women who've suffered miscarriage or stillbirth and do not share that sense of peace but rather continue to long for a successful pregnancy.

"Reconciling with that guilt really resonates for me," I confessed. "I'm emerging from it feeling relieved that a baby didn't happen. I trust that it wasn't the right time, or perhaps even the right partnership—whatever the case, it wasn't our child, and that's okay." I was speaking with a conviction I didn't know I had. Was bearing witness to Golda's assurance and resolve giving me, in turn, strength and courage? "I'm okay not getting pregnant." The rising pitch in my voice exposed my fragility.

Golda and I laughed. Like a pair of leather boots, with time, it would get more comfortable to walk the walk.

I took a deep breath and slowly exhaled while Golda nodded.

"I actually believe that," I said. "The dust is finally settling. I feel more grounded, like myself again."

Golda shook her head and leaned in to take my hand in her warm palms. "Whether we're in that uncertainty or peace about it not happening, there's still the frigging hormones and the loss of being pregnant. The fact that I got to deliver Tru adds another layer of mothering. Being a mom in one moment, and then not— *that* is miscarriage." She gave my hand an extra squeeze before letting go, then sank back into the couch. "So, I guess we can hold both."

"Sometimes I have to wonder," I said, "is this me telling myself it's okay or have I actually found peace and fulfillment?" The further I was from my miscarriage and the more women with whom I shared stories of loss, the clearer I became that this was right. Yet, some tensions remained. "I feel relief and, cognitively, I get that I shouldn't feel guilty, but . . ."

"Thank you for naming that relief," Golda said. "This is why you're listening to stories. Certainly for me, through your healing, I'm healing."

It was cathartic to hear her reassurances. Meta-cathartic.

I had no idea I would encounter someone like Golda when I suffered my loss or even the infertility. Here was the very woman Rae had envisioned—the presumably illusory forty-something who'd wanted a child, lost a pregnancy, and ultimately found peace without children. Now I understood why Rae had wanted to meet her, for Golda was helping me see that I, too, could embrace a childfree life. And all it took was sharing stories—an essential marker on my path to healing.

I asked Golda why she felt there wasn't more of an open dialogue around pregnancy loss.

"I have chills when you say that," she said, her body rippling upward. "Our parents' generation doesn't get why we publicize stuff like that on social media, but it's actually super healing for me to connect with others, whether in person or online, and be in sisterhood around this topic. Same thing with sexual misconduct and the whole #MeToo movement. I shared my miscarriage story on Facebook last April on the birth date of Truman. It was healing for other people, and I believe that's why it was such an easy 'yes' to talking to you: because we need to be sharing stories and normalizing pregnancy loss."

I asked Golda how she thought we might normalize the dialogue more effectively.

"I love your question and the possibility of it, but also, that's a big fucking hurdle." Golda's eyes searched around the room, then flicked back toward me. "You know those books for kids, like *Everyone Poops* or *The Gas We Pass*? Just like everyone farts, it's okay to have a miscarriage. Normalizing it through education, early on. The thing is, doctors usually don't know why it happened. Mothers and would-be mothers don't know. But *I* wanted to know why I miscarried."

Without a medical explanation readily available to her, Golda felt more validated in her belief that Truman had opted out. She emphasized that being childless didn't preclude her from being a mother; rather, she considers herself, and other women like us, "childless mothers." Once a mother—who had a growing fetus inside her, miscarried, and labored that once-growing being—always a mother.

I was curious to hear how Golda related motherhood to womanhood.

"Oh my gosh! I love being a woman!" she whispered, grabbing her breasts. "When I was pregnant, I felt very feminine. Hair's glowing, body's feeling voluptuous, and it's just so, 'Wow! I'm a woman!' So how *can* we hold these as separate?" She shook her curls off her shoulders and scanned her body. "I still have this voluptuous body, big breasts, and soft hair. I look in the mirror and love the beauty I see. I actually have a lot of masculine qualities, like hustling for my business and all that, but the physicality of being a woman feels very much present for me. When I hear people complain about getting their period, sure, I get it. But I'm like, 'Woohoo! I got my period!'" She paused and gave me a confused smile. "Am I even answering your question?"

"You are," I said as we laughed. "Whether actively mothering or not, you're still a woman in all your glory."

"Absolutely. Child or not . . . and period or not!" She smiled and mouthed, "Menopause."

Golda was right. I felt the gears of my brain shift, clicking and squeaking and grinding away, as I absorbed the many self-affirming lessons this journey, and these women, had taught me. I could and would celebrate my womanhood, my *humanity*—independent of motherhood, fertility, menstrual cycles, or other limiting factors. I was enough. We were enough. And we needed one another to help us recognize it and believe it.

"It's so important to have these conversations among women," Golda said. "We need to remember: we are not alone."

I was not alone. We carried each other through.

GLOSSARY

Clomid is a fertility drug used to stimulate egg production and promote ovulation.

D&C, dilation and curettage, is a surgical abortion procedure done in the first trimester to scrape away the womb lining.

D&E, dilation and evacuation, is a surgical abortion procedure done in the second trimester where the patient's cervix is dilated and suction is used to remove the fetus.

Endometriosis is an often painful disorder in which tissue similar to that which normally lines the inside of the uterus grows outside of it.

HCG, short for human chorionic gonadotropin, is a hormone secreted during pregnancy by the placenta which stimulates continued production of progesterone by the ovaries.

IUI, intrauterine insemination, referred to as donor or alternative insemination, is a procedure whereby sperm from a donor's collected semen are "washed" then injected into the uterus at the time of ovulation to support egg fertilization.

IVF, in vitro fertilization, is an assisted reproductive treatment wherein mature eggs are retrieved from ovaries and fertilized by sperm in a lab.

LEEP, Loop Electrosurgical Excision Procedure, is a treatment that prevents cervical cancer by using a small electrical wire loop to remove abnormal cervical cells.

Letrozole is a fertility drug used to induce ovulation and promote follicle growth.

Metformin is an oral medication to lower glucose and insulin levels; for women with PCOS, it enhances ovulation and regulates menstrual cycles.

Miscarriage is a loss before the 20th week of pregnancy. Approximately 80% of miscarriages take place within the first 12 weeks of pregnancy.

Misoprostol is an oral mediation used for abortion, medical management of miscarriage, induction of labor, cervical ripening before surgical procedures, and the treatment of postpartum depression.

Polycystic ovary syndrome is a treatable hormonal disorder affecting 10% of women of childbearing age. PCOS causes ovarian cysts and stunts the development of eggs released by the ovaries.

"Rainbow baby" refers to the child born after the metaphoric storm of miscarriage or stillbirth, who represents hope. A "sunshine baby" is the child born before a loss; an "angel baby," the loss.

Stillbirth is a loss after the 20th week of pregnancy.

Trisomy is the presence of a third chromosome in the body's cells instead of the normal two, causing developmental abnormalities.

END NOTES

1. Carla Dugas and Valori Slane, "Miscarriage." *StatPearls*, 2021, accessed August 30, 2021, https://pubmed.ncbi.nlm.nih. gov/30422585.

2. Craig P Griebel, et al. "Management of Spontaneous Abortion." *American Family Physician*, vol. 72,7 (2005): 1243-50. https://pubmed.ncbi.nlm.nih.gov/16225027.

3. David Denborough, "Traveling Down the Neuropathway: Narrative Practice, Neuroscience, Bodies, Emotions and the Affective Turn." *International Journal of Narrative Therapy and Community Work*, Vol. 3, 2019, 13-53. https://dulwichcentre.com. au/wp-content/uploads/2019/10/Journal-FULL-3-2019.pdf.

4. Kathryn R Grauerholz, et al., "Uncovering Prolonged Grief Reactions Subsequent to a Reproductive Loss: Implications for the Primary Care Provider." *Frontiers in Psychology*, vol. 12. May 12, 2021. https://www.ncbi.nlm.nih.gov/pmc/articles/PMC8149623.

5. Teri Pearlstein, et al., "Postpartum depression." *American journal of obstetrics and gynecology*, vol. 200,4 (2009): 357-64. https:// www.ncbi.nlm.nih.gov/pmc/articles/PMC3918890.

6. Elaine Webber and Jean Benedict, "Postpartum depression: A multi-disciplinary approach to screening, management and

breastfeeding support." *Archives of Psychiatric Nursing*, vol. 33,3 (2019): 284-289. https://pubmed.ncbi.nlm.nih.gov/31227081.

7. UN Women, "Intersectional feminism: what it means and why it matters right now," accessed January 11, 2021. https://www.unwomen.org/en/news/stories/2020/6/explainer-intersectional-feminism-what-it-means-and-why-it-matters. Inspired by Kimberlé W. Crenshaw. *On Intersectionality: Essential Writings*. 2017, The New Press, NY.

8. Trisomy 18 Foundation, "What is Trisomy 18?" accessed March 3, 2021, https://www.trisomy18.org/what-is-trisomy-18.

9. Fertility IQ, "Cost," accessed March 30, 2021, https://www.fertilityiq.com/topics/cost.

10. US Dept. of Health and Human Services Office on Women's Health, "Polycystic Ovary Syndrome" accessed August 31, 2021. https://www.womenshealth.gov/a-z-topics/polycystic-ovary-syndrome.

11. California Association of Realtors, "Historical Housing Data." Accessed on December 12, 2019, https://www.car.org/marketdata/data/housingdata; see also Kathleen Pender, "Bay Area Median Home Price Fell 2.3% Last Year, First Annual Drop Since 2011," *SF Chronicle*, January 17, 2020. https://www.sfchronicle.com/business/networth/article/Bay-Area-median-home-price-fell-2-3-last-year-14985353.php.

12. Dena T Smith et al. "Reviewing the Assumptions About Men's Mental Health: An Exploration of the Gender Binary." *American Journal of Men's Health*, vol. 12,1 (2018): 78-89. https://www.ncbi.nlm.nih.gov/pmc/articles/PMC5734543.

13. Betsy Cooper, "I'm Six Weeks Pregnant, and I'm Telling the World: Against the mandatory secret first trimester," *New York Times*, January 14, 2020, https://www.nytimes.com/2020/01/14/opinion/announcing-pregnancy-early.html.

14. National Organization for Rare Disorders (NORD), "Toxic Shock Syndrome," accessed August 31, 2021. https://rarediseases.org/rare-diseases/toxic-shock-syndrome.

15. Foundation for Women's Cancer, "Gestational Trophoblastic Disease (GTD)," accessed August 31, 2021. https://www.foundationforwomenscancer.org/gynecologic-cancers/cancer-types/gestational-trophoblastic.

16. Center for Disease Control (CDC), "Maternal Mortality," accessed August 31, 2021. https://www.cdc.gov/nchs/maternal-mortality/index.htm.

ACKNOWLEDGMENTS

I AM FOREVER GRATEFUL to the shining stars of this book for their courage and their trust, and to the countless women and men whose stories did not wend their way onto these pages, including family, friends, colleagues, and complete strangers who opened up to me. Without them, none of this would have been possible. And to those who have not shared their stories, I am equally grateful. Everyone has a unique and compelling story, expressed or not.

I never considered myself a storyteller, and I could not have written this book without the tough love and candor of my critiquing group: Caitlin, Neal, Catherine, Tammy, Rebecca, Libby, Emmy, Sheryl, and Bonnie. I'm grateful for their confidence and tireless cheerleading.

Thanks to the fabulous team of editors, project managers, and publicists at She Writes Press and BookSparks for believing in me. Thanks especially to Brooke Warner for her inspiration and guidance, and to Lauren Wise for keeping me on track.

Steve and Sarah and the beloved community of artists at the Wellstone Center in the Redwoods provided a much-needed sanctuary for developing my voice and structuring the book. I am grateful for their generosity and the serendipitous introduction to my dear friend Lee, whose seemingly effortless editing and unwavering support has made me both a better writer and a better human.

Thanks to Joe for his input and encouragement, even as we painfully parted ways. Thanks to my many friends for their enthusiasm, affirmations, and, at times, loving bewilderment for my having taken on this project. A special thanks to Jenny Sauer-Klein for her heart-felt introductions and sisterly support.

My family has been my refuge throughout my grief and my growth, and I am beyond fortunate for their love and our ever-deepening connection. Thanks to Katy and Diane for their friendship and to my brothers, Sam and Michael, for being feminist fathers and compassionate partners to these incredible women. What an absolute joy to be an aunt to their children and to know now, in my bones, that my family is already complete.

Lastly, thanks to mother Betsy, who continues to teach me about our capacity to love.